THE SINGLE MOST OVERLOOKED PROBLEM IN BACK PATIENTS

A Practical Three-Step Approach to Immediately Enhancing Patient Results, Increasing Practice Growth, and Improving Work Satisfaction

BY
Arjan Kuipers
DC, BSc, DACNB, FACFN, FEAC (Neurology)

CONTENTS

INTRODUCTION

LITTLE IS MORE FRUSTRATING THAN
A PATIENT PLAGUED BY PAIN WHOSE CONDITION
ISN'T RESPONDING TO YOUR TREATMENT.

**WOULD YOU BE RELIEVED TO KNOW
I MIGHT HAVE THE REMEDY YOU AND YOUR
PATIENT ARE SEEKING?**

Dear Fellow Practitioner,

In this report I will address two problems which go largely unnoticed that back patients in our care often face. If addressed properly, these two problems can be fairly easily overcome, greatly benefiting both you those in your care.

Perhaps it's best to start with the most uncomfortable problem needing to be addressed. It involves you and me and our unwillingness to change and see things in a broader perspective.

In other words, getting practitioners like us out of their comfort zones.

We must accept the fact that our current approach may *not* always be the best way to address the common problems encountered daily in our practices.

To accept this we will first have to get honest with ourselves.

In talking to colleagues I often hear the surprising results they have with their patients. It is not uncommon for me to hear others claim that up to 90% of their patients "get better" under their specific care.

"Wow," I think. "That's incredible."

But, let's get realistic. These are not typical results. I'm often led to wonder what these practitioners mean by "better". Is it better when their patients are in less pain? When they have less frequent back aches? *When those patients don't return to their clinics?*

I, for one, know that 90% of my patients don't get "better" with treatment. Maybe not even 50%.

But I know I'm doing everything I've been taught to do. So what's the trouble?

BEFORE CONTINUING: A CAVEAT

If you believe you belong to the select few chiropractors capable of reaching a 90% or more "betterment" rate from your patients, then I suggest it may be a waste of time for you to read this full report. **If, however, you feel you are in the group of chiropractors who are honest with themselves, read on.** If you are part of that second group, we share an ambition: we know we can't cure *all* our patients using standard methods, but we have a strong desire and believe there is a way to vastly improve our patients' quality of life in other ways.

If you are like me and you deeply desire to learn something new, something that can change your and your patients' lives and quality of life, this report will provide you with valuable advice on how to proceed with your practice and how to put some of the latest and most fascinating new medical knowledge to work for you.

I believe that, by the end of this report, you will better understand why it pays off to look beyond the standard bio-mechanical or pain-centred approach to back pain.

So, to start, the best question to ask yourself about your back patients is:

> *"Do most of my patients improve, or*
> *are they (and I) frustrated with*
> *what I can **and cannot** do for them?"*

MORE THAN JUST PATIENT CARE

In addition to improving your patients' condition(s), perhaps you want...

- *More personal satisfaction from your practice*
- *To do more for your patients*
- *Better results with your treatments*
- *More satisfied patients*
- *Patients who return with problems other than back pain*
- *Patients who truly trust you*
- *Patients who continually refer you*

And, if it were possible, would you also want to *grow your practice* in the process of *doing more for your patients?*

These are all good questions. And this report intends to assist you in achieving the things listed on the previous page.

What you will learn here is something most of us have overlooked or, frankly, categorically ignored. I'll outline steps you can take beginning today in order to improve your treatments, improve patient outcomes, improve their quality of life, and reduce the severity of their problems.

WHAT YOU SHOULD NEVER DO

This report isn't a cure all for your patients and your practice. While the claims I've made in the previous paragraph might sound like I'm offering a miracle means to making everything "better", I'm not. You should *never* say that. **You should never say to your patient, "I can help you *for sure* with this or that."** That's simply pretentious; any practitioner who claims they can fix any problem is putting their practice, their patients, and their livelihood at serious risk.

(If you don't agree with me, please stop reading! This report is NOT for you. Only people who can be honest with themselves will obtain any benefit from this publication.)

WHAT YOU SHOULD ALWAYS DO

Learn. Learn, learn, learn, and be open to learning even more. What did I say earlier? Our first challenge is to overcome:

OUR UNWILLINGNESS TO CHANGE AND SEE THINGS IN A BROADER PERSPECTIVE.

And, if you're open to it, I'm ready to teach you. You'll discover...

>   **...how to accomplish more** with your "standard" back, neck, and headache patients by attending to issues in their arms and legs other than the standard problem areas.

>   **...how to get better results from the "difficult" patients**, the ones who hesitate when you ask them for more details; who question you when you inquire beyond their back and neck problems; the ones who don't respond well to your treatment.

>   **...there are no new techniques to master** in order to improve outcomes for your patients.

>   **...that you do NOT have to spend more years and lots of money to master these new insights.**

>   **...the improved relationships applying this new knowledge will create with your patients** because you'll be able to better inform them, to explain more about their condition(s), and to respond more accurately to their more pointed questions and needs.

I have to be honest: knowing what I know—what I've included inside this report—has paid off and not just for my patients, but also for myself. The information you're about to learn has improved *my* practice, *my* job satisfaction, and how I feel overall about our wonderful profession.

FULFILL TWO REQUIREMENTS BEFORE CONTINUING

You have to *pay attention* and you have to be *willing to learn.* This report contains a lot of new material. It will give you a lot of things to think about and it'll be tempting to set it down to do research and check my discoveries against the most recent medical journals and publications at your disposal.

But it's imperative that you resist th at urge.

You need to read this report ONCE THROUGH IN ONE SITTING before stopping to do anything else. Give yourself time – maybe two solid hours – to read through it. Get rid of all the distractions. Turn off your phone(s). Put away your journals and turn off any other computers or electronic devices in the vicinity. **Sit in an isolated room if you have to.** Just make sure that you are not distracted! This is what I mean by "pay attention".

(People are much more distracted nowadays than at any other time in history, and it's not only due to electronics and technology invading our private space: we, as a human race, have taken multi-tasking too close to heart... we rarely sit and do one thing at a time. Doing only one thing at a time is actually *difficult* for many people!)

Take a moment to relax and open your mind and prepare for learning. Come to understand you will have questions; that things may not sound right at first and you'll want to fact check. *But, trust me: read the report through.* You'll find many of your questions are answered within these very pages.

Try to let go of mental and emotional distractions, too— upcoming appointments, to-do lists, anxiety, and other obligations—then grab a pen and paper and get ready to take plenty of notes because there are many gems you'll want to earmark for later.

And remember: this report may well be the eye-opener you've needed to get more out of your profession.

I hope you find here the knowledge you've long been seeking to grow your practice, improve your patients' care, and, overall, become a better chiropractor.

Yours in Health,

Arjan Kuipers,
DC, BSc, DACNB, FACFN, FEAC (Neurology)

CHAPTER 1

THE MOST OVERLOOKED PROBLEM

So, what's the big deal? What's this "single most overlooked problem in back patients"?

Before getting to that, I'd like to make something very, *very* clear: I'm not suggesting that I hold the one and only key to all the wisdom you'll ever need to succeed in your practice; I'm not claiming that there aren't other things that are *also* important.

But, if you keep up with today's worldwide medical literature, you'll realise that what I'm sharing with you is actually **one of the largest growing problems affecting of the world's population.** It's an issue that will continue to affect more and more patients in your daily practice.

And, trust me: of those you're already practicing on, there are a number of them currently suffering the effects of this much-neglected problem.

AT THE CENTRE OF OUR PROFESSION

This is one of those factors that we *should* address, but we don't. **It has to do with the nervous system.** And, historically, chiropractors claim to be masters of how the nervous system relates to the postural system.

Perhaps that's a bit boastful, saying chiropractors are the masters of understanding the nervous-postural relationship. Surely, we know a lot about back, neck, and related problems caused by subluxation, pinched nerves, or other conditions commonly considered "chiropractic issues", but we certainly don't know enough about the nervous system to be able to deal with other problems *caused by* the nervous system… right?

Wrong.

Most chiropractors do not look farther than the peripheral nervous system and the segmental effects their treatments have on that system. Alongside that, most chiropractors— both those new to the profession and those seasoned in their practice—maintain the concept that local spinal dysfunction, "pressure on nerves", causes problems, pain, and varied disease. Their greatest concern is relieving that troublesome pressure and, thus, alleviating pain and eventually curing the disease.

But, if it's that simple, if that's how the body works, why aren't more patients getting better? Why do patients have reoccurring problems, or problems that just *don't seem to go away,* no matter how many times that pressure is relieved or how many times they come to see you?

Because it's an old-fashioned way of practicing. This old view is one spawned from limited knowledge about the nervous system, *especially the brain.* And, unfortunately, most chiropractors don't know much about the nervous system other than the basic facts they have gleaned from chiropractic school.

Let's think deeper. Realise that **the nervous system I'm talking about consists 80% of the *central* nervous system—** the brain in particular—and that the brain governs most, if not all, of the other functions of the human body *including* the back, neck, and postural systems. *Next realise that you do not know enough about the central nervous system (CNS) to really claim that you affected it through standard chiropractic treatment.*

That's the reality.

SELF-EXAMINATION

Take a look at your practice. We all (myself included, at least at one time) maintain a high percentage of patients who experience the same, recurring problems despite treatment. Even more ridiculous, the truth is that patients who are experiencing *different* recurring problems are often treated in a similar way to *one another!* That's like...

...*a dentist using the same procedure for both a cavity and a loose tooth...*

...*or an optometrist issuing the same prescription for both near- and far-sighted patients...*

...*or an MD offering the same prescription for both a headache and a broken leg!*

Therefore, if other healthcare professions don't use the same treatment for different ailments, why do we?

Why is it that we aren't approaching the matters—both the recurring problems themselves *and* the different recurring problems—differently?

"INSANITY IS DOING THE SAME THING OVER AND OVER AND *EXPECTING A DIFFERENT RESULT.*"

-ALBERT EINSTEIN

Einstein's quote hits it right on the head: we're crazy if we think that the same treatment that didn't work last time (or the consecutive ten times prior) will work this time, or that we can use one treatment for a variety of different ailments.

We need to be honest with ourselves and accept the fact that, despite our training, **we may not be approaching our patients' problems in the best possible way.**

So the issue becomes one of moving past our formal chiropractic training and into a mode of self-training and re-examination of what we consider "standard" treatment.

And that's what I hope to accomplish by sharing this report with you.

The knowledge contained herein is strongly backed by the scientific community. Current and active medical studies are revealing more and more the role of the CNS in back pain, general pain problems, and larger pain and non–pain conditions.

To say it in fewer words:

What we are dealing with here is one of the biggest challenges in health care in this present day and age.

CHAPTER 2

THE CENTRE OF THE CENTRAL NERVOUS SYSTEM

In the previous chapter I mentioned that, while chiropractors are all too aware of the nervous system's relationship to pain and illness, we haven't yet put together that it's really the *central nervous system* which rules the functions we are trying to correct.

That's right: the brain. The brain and the influence it has on…

- *Pain*
- *Disease*
- *the Postural System*
- *Overall Health*

Whether you realise it or not (or accept it or not), the brain is central to the many problems in your daily practice. *Nay, it is the source of many of the problems in your daily practice!* If you think you can escape this fact, you're mistaken. And while we all know, intrinsically, that the brain is the centre of the nervous system—the system chiropractors are said to be "masters" of—we, as a healthcare profession, *have not bothered to learn more about it!*

Are you beginning to see the problem?

DAY-TO-DAY OBSERVATIONS

If you've been practicing for any length of time you'll likely have noticed a change in the population we're treating. If you haven't taken notice, **now is the time to contemplate differences between your patients at the start of your practice and your patients now.** It's also a good time to start making a habit of noting those differences in your patient files.

What differences am I talking about? To name a few:

1. *We're seeing more people with dementia.* As a greater percentage of the population is under suspicion that there is something going on with their minds, the brain's decline in function may indicate the early stages of Alzheimer's disease.

2. *We're seeing more children* and *adults with Autism Spectrum Disorder.* Since the DSM-V psychiatric handbook has been introduced, Autism Spectrum Disorder nowadays generally is used interchangeably with classical Autism, a Pervasive Developmental Disorder Not Otherwise Specified (PPD-NOS) as Asperger's Syndrome.

3. *We're seeing more children with ADHD, including ADD variants.* In addition to the absolute increase in numbers, more and more girls, adults, and parents of children with a known diagnosis are themselves being diagnosed with ADHD.

4. *We're seeing more people with traumatic brain injuries.* This is very, very important for chiropractics. Traumatic brain injury is *huge;* it can lead to bodily *compensations* that have an enormous impact on the postural system, as well as on spinal or overall skeletal health.

5. *And we're seeing many patients with a general decline in brain function* for three simple reasons: (a) they are not educating themselves, i.e. they aren't stimulating and growing their cognitive abilities; (b) they are not changing the way they approach their emotions; and (c) they are not *moving their bodies* (exercising), which has a huge influence on the health of the brain.

You'll notice these are all brain-related conditions: dementia, Autism Spectrum, ADHD. And not just "brain-related", but, more specifically, brain declinative.

That's why the rest of this report will focus on the brain's influence over the postural system as well as the brain's influence on the spine and pain. And, as previously mentioned, most of us haven't dealt with the brain or nervous system in any way other than the "standard treatments" we've applied to the spine or the actual skeleton.

And remember that the spine and skeleton are under control of the brain. *So, if we don't change the brain, we'll* **never** *truly change the spine or skeleton.*

That's not to say we can't have some impact on the brain by treating the postural system. Treatment of the postural system *can* have an impact upon the brain. Surely, we can realign the body and create new musculo-skeletal "memory" within the brain. But that's a very slow, time consuming process.

Wouldn't you like to know of other ways you can help the process along a little faster?

If you answered "yes", you're in the right place! As a healthcare professional, you *should* want to know a little bit more! If you answered "yes", *that means you're on the right track to changing the way you think about your profession.*

Therefore, proceed confidently! Know that by reading through and absorbing the knowledge of this report you'll be able to understand the brain-postural relationship 10%, maybe even 20% better. **You'll be that much more equipped and that much more capable of improving the health of your patients' brains.** You WILL greatly improve the treatment results of your patient population and, therefore, you WILL be able to help them achieve the improved quality of life they've so been seeking.

ATTACKING THE PROBLEM

Now we know that the biggest problem is brain decline. Alzheimer's, dementia, and childhood developmental disorders such as autism and ADHD are all treated as diseases with different causes when, in reality, they're all related to unidentified and undiagnosed brain decline and dysfunction.

And, while brain decline is the biggest problem—OUR biggest problem—it's also the grey area of brain function.

If something immediately goes wrong with the brain (such as swelling, bleeding, or other critical injury) we go see an allopathic practitioner, i.e. the MD, the doctor in the hospital. That's their turf: urgency. That's when they know the best thing to do.

But everything before that critical state is *dysfunction.* And dysfunction is where we, as chiropractors, can help, because whether or not a person ever sees an allopathic practitioner for immediate critical care, most people will experience brain decline or dysfunction sometime in their life. There are probably only a handful of patients in your clinic—a select lucky few—who do not or will not suffer from this problem. That's reality.

WHETHER OR NOT THEY
EVER SEE AN MD FOR
IMMEDIATE CRITICAL
CARE, MOST PEOPLE WILL
EXPERIENCE BRAIN DECLINE
OR DYSFUNCTION
SOMETIME IN THEIR LIFE.

The rest of the report will teach you how to detect these dysfunctions, or at least begin to start recognising them. *You'll begin to learn how to deal with these problems in a logical and clinical way, in a way that is an extension of your already existing practice.* You won't even have to put yourself through more years of formal education or spend more money to master these techniques and to be able to start dealing with these problems. But you will need to achieve those two prerequisites I mentioned earlier: **paying attention and having a willingness to learn.**

CHAPTER 3

MY BACKGROUND

We know from basic medical study that the brain's job is to keep you alive in the most efficient way possible. For example, by handling dangers in the environment such as viruses and allergens; to oversee bodily functions such as digestion and perspiration; and even to aid in psychological wellness by helping (or hindering) memory. The ability of the brain to be able to do all this, 365/24/7, is determined by the existence, or lack, of three influences:

OXYGEN

NUTRITION

ENVIRONMENTAL STIMULATION

Surprisingly, most health-related professions have a complete lack of understanding on how the brain works, how it flourishes, and how it is kept in optimal condition. **This gives us ample opportunity to start changing how we and everybody else looks at chiropractics.** We can move from being simply reactive—treating backaches, neck pains, headaches—and be *proactive.*

If we are claiming to be the profession which deals with spinal and skeletal problems—ultimately, with problems in the postural system—then we'd better shape up and learn more about the brain!

Compensation Confusion

One thing to note about the brain is that it is very good at providing compensations for injury or disease. For example, if vision is diminished or lost altogether, the brain will make up for the deficiency by amplifying the other senses. It's actually a fully automated and very miraculous system.

And, like so many things that are automated, people take it for granted. Most people won't even realise when the system has made a compensative change. If they *do* realise it, they'll often not think to mention it to a healthcare practitioner because, to them, the problem is "fixed". Even fewer patients will know of the compensation, know they should share it, but then decline to mention it for pride, embarrassment, or other reasons.

And, if YOU don't pay attention to your patient(s), then YOU won't notice these changes either.

And if you don't notice the changes, you won't be able to help your patients attain a better level of health. And, remember, it's not just spinal health we're talking about, but *overall health*.

Why I'm Passionate about Brain Function

Before we get any further, I think it's only fair to explain why I'm so passionate about the topic of brain wellness and its relationship to postural function and overall health.

When I grew up, my mother suffered a series of accidents—car accidents and slips in which she knocked her head—and the result was debilitating. Literally.

A couple of times a week she would experience strange attacks. She would be unable to walk. Her speech would slur. Her ability to react to the environment would deteriorate. She would lie on the floor or on a bed or on a couch, wherever it was that she had collapsed, and would shake her upper body, her arms, and her neck, and her body would disturbingly extend while suffering through these episodes.

It wasn't epilepsy, but it certainly looked like it.

Over the years, her condition worsened. She was able to work in between the episodes, but only because a chiropractor managed her situation. *All the other healthcare professionals we saw claimed there was nothing wrong with her.* All the scans, blood tests, and other examinations had not resulted in any conclusion. According to the "regular" medical world, there was no condition that could cause this. They diagnosed her "untreatable".

It was ludicrous. For an MD to know what she was going through, to know what her symptoms were, to know her bodily pain and anguish, to visibly *see* the problem… then to say, "There's nothing wrong."

That is *absolutely* unacceptable.

Especially when, strangely enough, she was able to find relief from her situation through treatments to her postural system. A chiropractor did something to her postural system—some kind of adjustment—and she would sometimes very quickly, sometimes a little bit slower, find relief from her epileptic-like episode. If the chiropractor didn't treat her, the episode would continue on and on.

For me, a teenager at the time, this chiropractor's treatment was magic. And, because the situation with my mother was a critical part of my life—not only that she was my mother, a great influencer in my life, but that her condition changed how our family lived and thought about the world—when time came to decide what kind of profession I wished to be in I only saw two choices before of me: standard medicine or chiropractics.

And, after working for a year as a janitor, I made up my mind: I was going to learn how to deal with my mother's situation. I was going to address medical issues at their core and solve problems, not put myself into situations where I'd have to deem illnesses "untreatable".

I was going to become a chiropractor.

So, 25 years ago I went to England and studied at A.E.C.C., the Anglo-European College of Chiropractic. I became a chiropractor; I thought, I hoped, to learn how to effectively deal with my mother's situation. Unlike others in my class, I wasn't led to chiropractic school because I wanted to know how to treat back pain or neck pain or headaches. *I wanted to learn how the brain and the body interacted.* Above all, I wanted to help my mother so she could finally rid herself of her condition, whatever it was.

Though I learned a lot at A.E.C.C., I was somewhat disappointed with the course and content of my studies.

As you all well know, there's a lot to be learned in chiropractic school, but very little of the curriculum deals directly with *how the brain and the body interact* and *how to treat those interactions when they go wrong.* So for the first two years of practicing I was, to say the least, frustrated because I still didn't know how to deal with these attacks my mother had. Other than at a very, very basic level, I still wasn't able to understand what was going on between her brain and her body.

But sometimes from frustration springs new ambition. Sometimes frustration can cause you to re-think a situation and can spur you on to improve yourself.

Through my then-colleague (and boss and friend), Roland Blaauw, I was put into contact with Frederick Carrick, who had started teaching functional neurology to chiropractors.

Through those functional neurology courses I was able to decipher my mother's brain-body communications. I came to understand why my mother's symptoms were occurring; why they'd started; why they happened in the first place; what the root problem was; and, ultimately, how to treat her.

WHY WE'RE RIGHT FOR THE JOB

While my mother's treatment and medical success is the highlight of (and reason for) my career, I'd like to step back and take a broader view of what her success really means for us, for chiropractors.

I want you to understand a bit more about how YOU can affect the brain. I want you to know what this knowledge means to the patients we're seeing more and more of each day (as a refresher, re-read that list *here*). Finally, I want you to understand why it is that

CHIROPRACTORS ARE MORE SUITED TO TREATING THE BRAIN'S PROBLEMS
THAN MANY OTHER TYPES OF PRACTITIONERS.

But, to explain how this knowledge relates to all of us, let me backtrack to my story again:

After I solved the mystery of my mother's condition, I was feeling great. My knowledge was benefitting *all* my patients, not just my mother, and *I felt more able as a healthcare professional to treat things my colleagues couldn't,* or, rather, didn't know they could, treat. But that was only the beginning.

It was shortly after attending those neurology courses that I began seeing children in my practice with learning, developmental, and behavioural problems. Eventually I more or less specialized in this particular type of patient.

Along with this new specialization came new frustrations. After finding treatment for my mother's condition, I felt I knew a lot about the brain and the postural system. **But, with these children, the heartbreak started all over again.** It wasn't long before I realised that my current knowledge wasn't enough. I didn't know enough—even after solving my great mystery—in order to help improve the lives of these children with learning and behavioural problems.

Like before, when the new frustrations piled up, my thirst for answers grew ever stronger.

Currently, I hold a neural developmental specialization because of my knowledge of the brain. I'm able to help children who have neural behavioural disorders, like Autism, ADHD, learning disabilities (e.g. dyslexia), or developmental and motor skills problems. I better understand what I can do *as a chiropractor* for these children. I can improve the quality of their lives. And they don't have to just see an MD in an intimidating hospital, travel to a far-off specialty clinic, be relentlessly tested by neurological specialists, or take scary pharmaceuticals in order to have their lives improved.

It's just me, a chiropractor, in a comfortable office with no drugs, needles, or special equipment. Just me, and their parents, in a safe place.

I recently authored a book on ADHD and Autism entitled *Help! My Child has ADHD/Autism! The Life-Changing Insights Most Experts Still Don't Use.* It's the first in a series which illustrates my knowledge of and experience with the brain–postural system connection. This new knowledge, in unison with my studies in chiropractic and functional neurology, makes it possible for me to treat beyond a symptom. To parents of ADHD and Autistic children, I can…

…provide **COMFORT** by explaining what's happening in their children's brains and bodies…

...provide **REASSURANCE** by explaining what they can realistically expect from the regular, often limited, "standard medicine" approach...

...give them **POWER** by showing them what they can do themselves...

...offer them **KNOWLEDGE** on a more basic level about:
- what we (as a healthcare community) know and don't know about the brain,
- how the brain influences the body, and
- what external factors can influence and effectively *change* the brain.

Where before these parents of ADHD and/or Autistic children had suffered the let-down of false hopes, the anxiety of helplessness, and the overall disappointment of standard medicine, I was able to give them a firm footing and a solid—and true!—reason to be optimistic.

With their cooperation, I was (and am) able to brighten the lives of many children who otherwise had run out of places to turn.

The thing the parents often found most surprising: I was a "mere" chiropractor, *not* an MD!

SECONDARY BENEFITS

In addition to being able to treat a variety of ails with my newfound knowledge—from standard neck and back pains to behavioural, developmental, and learning disorders—I noticed **treatment required fewer visits with my patients.** It's rare for me to see any patient more than 2, 3 times in a week at the most. Even in the most acute cases, that number is excessive. (Don't worry, I'm not the type to see a patient one or two times and then wave them off as "cured". I strongly believe in patient management.)

Another beauty of learning the brain-postural connection is that **I could make better predictions about treatments.** I was learning along the way what worked best, what signs to look for, which symptoms were important and which weren't. In essence, I was fine-tuning my attentiveness, that skill that is so critical to determining and correctly diagnosing your patients. (While I don't believe anyone can accurately predict the right treatment for every patient, every time, and even though I openly admit I can't help ALL patients with increased brain-postural knowledge, those are issues beyond what this report addresses.)

But the greatest benefit was that my patients who I had considered "cured" came back, and not in the way you'd expect. That's right! **They came back with *other* problems.** They understood that, because I knew more than the average chiropractor, I had the capacity to help them with problems where medical (allopathic) doctors had failed.

"PATIENTS WHO I'D
TREATED CAME BACK,
**AND NOT IN THE WAY
YOU'D EXPECT."**

This can be you. You can be the one people come to for ails other practitioners have deemed mysterious or incurable. You can be the one they'll go to for ordinary things and those things out of the ordinary. In some cases, for those patients who are tired (or wary) of drugs' side effects and warnings, you could be their option for a non-pharmaceutical, safer, and longer-lasting treatment.

My practice has evolved into a large clinic with a lot of loyal patients, and I know its success is largely due to my passion about the brain's functions.

I had no doubts when I set out to learn more about the brain-postural connection that I'd be better able to affect those individuals who came directly to me and my clinic.

However, little did I know that I'd be presented with opportunities to help people in faraway places, in cities, states, and countries outside my known circles.

FAR-REACHING ADVANTAGES

I was recently invited speak on a current hot topic. One of the biggest newspapers in Holland approached me about participating in a story about the danger of energy drinks. My part: energy drinks and the effects they have on the brain.

That's why they contacted me. Because of my brain knowledge.

Who knows where that article went, how many times and places it was published, or how many eyes were able to read it and be influenced by it. Regardless of those answers, I felt honoured that a huge influencer in the media was seeking my expertise.

When you begin applying your learned brain knowledge—the knowledge you'll reap from this report—to your practice, word will get out. **Word of mouth is still the single most powerful advertising method in the world,** even following television, the Internet, billboards, print ads, or mailers.

When your patients talk about you to others, your practice will begin to change in more ways than you can imagine.

So that's what this knowledge has brought me. I not only help the patients in my clinics better, but I also help people I've never even met through writing, lecturing, and through interviews to the media. You'll be surprised to find out just how many people want to know how the brain and the body interact, and how they can apply that knowledge *in their daily lives* to start feeling better.

PEOPLE WANT TO KNOW
HOW THE BRAIN AND
BODY INTERACT,
AND HOW THEY CAN
**APPLY THAT KNOWLEDGE
IN THEIR DAILY LIVES TO
START FEELING BETTER.**

BUILDING BUSINESS

Like any other business, chiropractors' practices run off simple economics: a basic system of supply and demand. You have a service to supply that is balanced and kept in check depending on how much the population demands it. **So if you could add to your business something that everyone wants... why wouldn't you do it?** That's why this report isn't something you should take for granted.

Just knowing how much people everywhere *want to know about the brain-body connection ought to be one of the chief motivations and reasons for why you need to carefully read through and absorb this information.*

If for no other reason, there's a huge profit to be made by learning about the brain. I know for a fact that most doctors like us have a fairly good knowledge of the brain; they know the basics of the influence of the brain on the body and of the standard regulatory mechanisms it dictates.

But what they don't know is...

What the information really means;

How to use that information to **influence** *patients and their* **practice;**

How to **recognise problems** *that might otherwise only be detected by a few, hard-to-access specialists; and*

How to **tend to those problems without drugs,** *surgery, or questionable "standard" healthcare practices.*

And these are the things you're going to learn.

CHAPTER 4

BRAIN GOVERNMENT

Now that I've given you both a background and multiple reasons for carefully reading through this report, let's get into the more exciting details: the knowledge itself.

STARTING FROM THE BASICS

We'll begin with three truths.

1. The brain governs the spine.
2. The brain governs your postural system.

And, this third fact may shock you:

3. The spine is not controlled exclusively by segmental reflexes.

Yes, the back (i.e. the spine) is not only governed by segmental reflexes. This means that when you do something to the spine it has an effect on the brain and also that the spine—spinal health, spinal controls—is governed by what's happening in the brain.

In other words:

For the back and brain, communication goes both ways.

Accepting this new, two-way street approach to the brain and back has the potential for changing your entire practice. (In all honesty,

I hope it does!) If you start thinking differently about the work that you do, you'll see if differently; you'll see that *what you do to the spine, to the spinal column, affects basic brain functions,* and that any slight change can have a profound effect on the development and healing of someone's nervous system.

Where we have traditionally learned in chiropractic school about pressure on the nerves and how that pressure negatively effects the body... well, that's child's play compared to what's really happening.

And knowing that the information we've been given has been "dumbed down" for us also means we need to start asking ourselves a pretty serious question:

ARE WE REALLY THE EXPERTS— *THE ONES WHO KNOW THE MOST ABOUT THE NERVOUS SYSTEM* —THAT WE CLAIM TO BE?

In reality, the answer is "no". No, we aren't. It's a hard truth to swallow, but if we're going to get better we need to accept that fact. *We simply DO NOT know the most about the nervous system.* But when we are given an opportunity to improve—when we're given a chance to see how the brain and the spine interact, how brain health affects posture, orientation of the body, how it controls pain—we, as a profession, need to take it.

And that's what it is I'm talking about: increasing your awareness and teaching you how to begin with the fundamentals you already know and just slightly modifying your treatments in order to truly, and marvellously, control the communication between brain and spine, mind and body.

In the Beginning...

Have you ever wondered how it is that we stand upright? You know from previous studies that it isn't due to pure construction, the myriad muscles, tendons, capsules, bones, and discs that together form the body. And it certainly isn't the mere *existence* of the postural muscles that keep us upright, either.

Do you know how the deep spinal muscles—the core of your postural system, the muscles that stabilize all other muscles—are activated? Have you ever wondered about that? Or, like many, have you simply taken that knowledge for granted?

Well, it's time to look closer.

Think back to your neuroanatomy classes in chiropractic school. Remember, then, that it's the *Area Acoustica* of the brainstem that works to keep us standing. This area is activated by medial parts of the cerebellum (or frontal lobe), which in turn receives their direction from the deep spinal muscles and the rest of the postural system.

And remember that it's these same deep spinal muscles which are directly related to the eye muscles and the control of the eye muscles. (More on this later.)

Essentially:

There is ONE column of nerve cells which activate both the eye muscles and deep spinal muscles.

And if that column of nerve cells is damaged or diseased, we then have a problem with balance and standing upright.

Have you thought deeply about the relationship between balance and vision, eye muscles and spinal muscles? Do you know what other systems in the brain influence this delicate harmonisation?

When you start understanding that you'll really begin to see how the brain governs spinal function and how the proverbial wool has been pulled over our eyes. Unfortunately, that breadth of knowledge reaches beyond the scope of this report.

But, aside from that, just remember this:

The deep spinal muscles keeping a person erect are
under constant control of mechanisms in the brainstem,
which are under control of
higher cortical functions within the two hemispheres.

Spatial awareness and the body's ability to quickly react through muscular tension in order to adapt to the changing environment you move in is vital to normal spinal health. If spatial awareness

systems are not functioning
optimally and are out of
balance, that imbalance has
a profound impact on the
ability of the spine to adapt to
situations, to stabilize all the
other muscular functions. It
effects the muscles' abilities to
flex, react, and heal; muscular
control is lost in the shoulders,
pelvis, legs, neck, and in the movement of the head.

Spatial Awareness
The ability to consciously
understand the relationship
of objects in one's
surroundings as it relates to
one's own form.

It must be understood that imbalance in the spatial awareness systems are all due to improper operations in the brain caused by injury, disease, or dysfunction.

SPATIAL AWARENESS
IS VITAL TO
NORMAL SPINAL HEALTH.

I want to give you a real life example of just how you can improve overall health by paying attention to—and then treating—an imbalance in spatial awareness.

It's a chiropractor's common experience that a patient's recurring problem cannot always be explained away by what is viewed on a body scan or x-ray, or with any of the "normal" and "regular" orthopaedic and chiropractic testing that we have been taught to do.

In cases such as that, it may serve you well to consider that there might be something wrong with the control systems *other than* problems with strictly organic dysfunction. **Consider that it may be a systemic dysfunction,** that there might be [an]other underlying disease causing the trouble.

And this is also a very good time to show how, when you start to routinely treat patients, it's easy to overlook other problems that are present and how that oversight may interfere with appropriate reconditioning and recovery; how, if not addressed, will put you in a situation where a patient will not come back and go elsewhere to seek other help★, even if you have been able to help this patient over a long period of time on several occasions.

CASE STUDY: MARY

Mary[1] was your typical patient: a woman in her fifties complaining of pelvic pain. I'd treated her over the past two decades on a number of occasions for back and shoulder pains and my treatments before had helped her enough that she was confident I could help her again.

This time she came in complaining about pains around the pelvic girdle. When I did my physical examination I found no inflammation in the connective tissues or muscles. As protocol required, I asked her about her condition.

She said she had problems walking, that she would fatigue easily. This was no small thing, as Mary was a frequent and passionate long-distance walker. She explained how her stride had shortened; she simply couldn't make the same stride as she had before. She said that, when she fatigued, she would get pains in her upper legs. She also admitted that her cognition had decreased. She wasn't able to hold her concentration. Therefore, she wasn't reading as much as she used to; *she wasn't learning and keeping her mind occupied as much as she used to.*

I reluctantly admit that on that particular occasion, on the initial consultation for Mary's pelvic girdle pain, I was in a hurry. I didn't slow down, didn't ask enough about what was really going on. I focused on the local problems to pelvic pains, the walking problems. I did "my thing". *I listened to her complaints and moved forward with my standard treatment, the same treatment as I had used on her before.* I expected her to respond to the treatment as she had in the past. I was acting crazy.

★*Recall my concern over the "better" 90%. If those doctors are assuming non-returning patients simply don't return because they are cured, instead of considering that the patient was disappointed and went elsewhere... my! What an assumption, indeed!*

---

1 Name changed to maintain patient confidentiality.

But I found out on her follow-up appointment that her condition hadn't improved.

My curiosity perked.

It didn't take but a moment to see the mistake I'd made the first time around. I realised the trap I'd fallen into that so many of us are bound to experience and repeat: I hadn't listened.

On Mary's follow-up I made it a point to sit with her and really listen to what she had to say. We sat down. **She told me that she hadn't improved, that she might even be worse.** She could walk even less. She had continued pain around her pelvis.

I felt there was more, so I pressed on.

She explained that the pains in her legs and around her pelvis had developed over a period of weeks, if not months. From there she had started walking less and less, *activating her body less and less*. And, because she was so used to being able to go long distances, being able to go only a short way was *emotionally trying*. She also felt that her posture had changed; she had begun to stoop a little.

And, the most frustrating symptom: she had a constant mental fogginess. She just felt she was out of balance sometimes, both mentally AND physically.

I made her walk a few steps for me. I noticed that the distance between her thighs had widened a little from what it had previously been. Her posture had definitely changed. She'd gone into ante-flexion, into a stooped posture, causing her breathing to be shallow because her lungs couldn't fully expand.

I examined closer and performed some specific neurological examinations. I discovered her eye functionality had decreased, so much so that she couldn't even do some of the tests. *Her balance was very unsteady when I was examining her eye functionality.*

Next she mentioned she had just come out of a very emotionally tiring period. She was in the middle of moving; there had been some problems in the family; she had felt extremely stressed for some time.

After listening, it all became clear: Mary didn't have a *body* problem. She had a *brain* problem.

DIAGNOSIS: BRAIN

So we went back to the basics, those three essential elements of optimal brain function:

OXYGEN

NUTRITION

ENVIRONMENTAL STIMULATION

Perhaps she thought it silly, but I knew we had to re-teach her body how to do certain things.

First: oxygenation. I re-taught her how to breathe properly. We used some chiropractic techniques to improve her breathing, to improve her posture in order to give her lungs room to expand and help bring oxygen to her nervous system, to her *whole* system.

Second: nutrition. I gave her advice on how to eat more properly, especially in regard to more green vegetables. In talking digestion and diet, we came to realise her digestive system was experiencing problems, too. We helped that with some nutritional supplements.

Third: environmental stimulation. I gave her advice on specific brain supplements to take, like *Omega 3's with high DHA content* and the like, to help increase neurological function and rid her of mental fogginess. By omitting her "brain fog", her concentration would return, making reading, learning, and other mental stimulation exercises (including physical exercises), pleasurable again.

THE RESULTS ARE PROOF

Even though I didn't use manual chiropractic techniques on her pelvis, I only saw Mary twice. Following our second appointment, **Mary adhered to my advice and reaped her reward**: she experienced a significant improvement of her situation within four weeks of making the lifestyle changes I'd suggested (e.g. supplements, diet, posture).

It became very clear to both Mary and I that the small lifestyle changes and the changes in oxygenation of her body made a huge difference to her health. Though I was "only" a chiropractor, I'd done more than give her "standard" chiropractic treatment.

I'd changed her life experience.

Mary's situation isn't unique. Her situation could have happened anywhere, in any chiropractic office in any place in the world. As I said, she was a typical patient, one of many like her whom I saw and still see on a regular basis. *She is the typical patient we all see, the patient who won't respond to normal treatment, who only requires us to change our mode of thinking just slightly in order to heal them.* What made Mary different is that, where many patients usually neglect to inform, she was more than willing to share ALL her symptoms with me, even the ones that didn't seem to be symptoms.

She gave me the clues, and I followed the trail.

And that's what we need to do as a profession: be brain detectives. In order to truly take hold of our claim as nervous system experts we need to take the extra step, grab hold of those extra clues, so we can stand out from all the other healthcare professions which deal in the business of alleviating back and other types of pain.

CHAPTER 5

FOLLOW THE ANT

Now I'd like you to consider a basic three-step approach. This isn't something I came up with on my own, nor is it something that I'm able to patent or will even try to. It's just plain and simple, logical thinking encapsulated in an easy-to-remember acronym: ANT.

And when you learn this approach, you'll wonder how you ever practiced without it.

(I'll issue my short warning again: if you do not want to change, you don't think it's worth the effort or you're not going to even try it, then please don't waste your time.)

A IS FOR AWARENESS

Before doing anything—before deciding upon a treatment protocol or even deciding what the real trouble is with your patient—you need to first *have and maintain awareness* of two explicit truths:

- The brain and the postural system share an intimate relationship.
- Asking the right questions is the only way to get the information you need from your patients for proper diagnosis and treatment.

In regard to the first fact, *scientific literature will show this to be true.* The problem is with chiropractics: the way we've been applying our learned knowledge to our patients works contrary to scientific finding. We have adopted the [bad] habit of looking at the postural system, motorics, cognition, or emotions *separately*, when we should be looking at them as a singular system.

If you see how the brain evolves and how it develops, it's all one and the same system. The motorics of your body, cognition, and emotions are parallel systems, intimately related. This total-body approach includes taking into consideration the immune system, digestion, circulation, mood, and many other bodily functions.

They grow together. They're wired together.

Why on earth, then, did we uncouple them? Who started this tradition of looking at behaviour or cognition or emotional control or motorics singularly?

THE WAY WE'VE BEEN
APPLYING KNOWLEDGE TO OUR
PATIENTS WORKS
**CONTRARY TO SCIENTIFIC
FINDING.**

In regard to the second fact, your patients don't know what you need to know. Furthermore, you must be aware that even if you know someone, even if you've treated them before once or even many times, *if you don't ask the right questions you'll never know if something is going on with their brain.* You need to know about accidents they've had or problems (even minor ones!) with their cognition, past and present. You need to know their learning patterns, how clear they think, or if they've experienced any recent or recurring illnesses. (If you don't look at the immune system, you may not be aware that there are problems that hugely influence their postural health, their spinal health, or their pain.)

So awareness of problems with the brain and the central nervous system in relation to the spine is the *first* step toward accurate identification and, therefore, proper treatment.

NEUROLOGICAL TESTING

The actual physical work begins after you've identified the problem. That is, the chiropractic, neurological, and physiological examination of the patient.

Start looking at how the brain functions and you start recognising that small changes in the brain can have profound effects on the motorics of the body. And quite often not even the most obvious motorics like leg movement, because that is only a very, very small part of what the brain does, but very small things, like the eye's reflexogenic connections, which I'll address more in-depth later. When you begin to recognise these things—both large and small motorics issues—then you'll start deciphering the broken brain-postural (spinal) communication that your patient is experiencing as pain.

TREATMENT IS THE CURE

Following the neurological testing step, we need to fix the brain-postural communication problem by either:

1. *Improving the brain's health (more aptly, the brain's ability to heal itself;*
2. *Improving the brain's capacity [to deal with spinal problems]; or*
3. *Decreasing the spinal problems in ways other than by standard chiropractic treatment.*

Together these three elements—awareness, neurological examination, and treatment—form the ANT we need to follow.

CHAPTER 6

AWARENESS

Let's take a closer look at expanding and maintaining our awareness and identification of brain dysfunction and disease.

SMASHING ASSUMPTIONS

People regularly assume that when something is wrong with the brain the condition will be very obvious; we expect to be able to see it from a mile away. **Surely, everyone can recognise brain problems!** We assume a person with a troubled brain will need delicate care from a highly specialized allopathic doctor and needs to be seen both in the hospital for severe treatments and/or by the family physician on a regular basis.

But this "cover all" approach is completely wrong. We need to learn to separate disease from dysfunction.

BRAIN DYSFUNCTION ≠ BRAIN DISEASE

In most cases, the brain's function can decline with hardly any notice at all. It can be a slow, easing process which happens over a long period of time. There is no brain *disease*—no tumor, inflammation, or viral infection, to name a few—but there is some dysfunction there.

And this is where YOU come in. This is where you have to pay attention, because those patients with the dysfunction—*not the disease*—are the ones you'll see in your practice.

The worst assumption you can make as a healthcare professional is assuming your patient's brain is in good health. Even people who work in a high-functioning job or profession can experience brain decline and, because they're working in a high-functioning profession, they're able to mask the problem a lot longer than patients working low-paid, low-functioning jobs that do not require much mental activity (e.g. fast food, retail, low-end or repetitive manual labour). So be aware that ALL your patients may have brain health that's on the decline.

BEING A BRAIN DETECTIVE

Now that we know never to assume good neurological health in a patient, we need to know how to detect if something is wrong with your patient's brain.

When considering brain health assessment, keep in mind what I've said before: chiropractors are in a better position than most healthcare professionals to examine what's going on in the brain.

Why is that?

Well, we know there are specific brain questionnaires a healthcare professional can have a patient complete. And, by all means, do so! Those questionnaires are designed to detect the early stages of dementia or Alzheimer's, or even point to the possibility of tumours that have cognitive or emotional consequence. So, if the tools are there, use them.

WE ARE IN A BETTER
POSITION THAN MOST
HEALTHCARE
PROFESSIONALS TO
**EXAMINE WHAT'S GOING
ON IN THE BRAIN**

Traditionally, allopathic doctors rely partly on visual cues but heavily on diagnostic tests that are either timely, expensive, or both. Some examples of these tests involve blood panels, urine and stool samples, biopsies, MRI and CAT scans, and the like.

But, our practice is very visual and kinaesthetic. That's what makes us different.

As chiropractors, we *watch* people: how they sit, how they stand, how they walk; how their nervous system is communicating (or not) with their muscles or muscle groups; how their digestion is operating and if there are headaches present or not.

As a chiropractor, it's natural for you to look at what's happening with the motorics of the body—with the motor output of the brain and with the signals the brain sends to the body—both to the voluntary motor controls and the autonomic nervous system, which controls organ function. For example, like any other motor function, blood pressure is under the influence of the brain, so vascular tonicity (the tonicity of your muscles around your vessels) is under the influence of your brain's function.

Because our profession so heavily relies on visualization and immediate diagnoses, we are better able to look at the visual motor consequences and make sense of them.

And in order to do so accurately—and to also be able to explain your reasoning to your patient(s)—it's very likely that you'll have to expand greatly upon the chiropractic knowledge you have now and incorporate *brain knowledge* into your expertise.

Thus, the best way to look at what's happening in the brain is to look at the motor consequences, because motorics are the result of every communication coming into and out of the brain.

And the purpose of a motoric evaluation is to, ultimately, complete a full neurological examination of your patient(s).

CHAPTER 7

NEUROLOGICAL EXAMINATION

In this chapter we'll approach just HOW to assess the health of the brain through neurological examination. That is the next point, after all: the 'N' in ANT.

DETAILS ARE EVERYTHING

So what motor consequences, exactly, are we talking about? I believe the better question is

WHAT ARE THE MOTOR CONSEQUENCES
WE CAN *SEE* WHEN THE BRAIN IS
EXPERIENCING DYSFUNCTION?

When a person has brain trauma due to an injury or compensation illness (for example, from an acute vestibular inflammation resulting in acute balance problems to which the brain/body had to stabilise), *the compensation and trauma still exist even though the injury or illness has "healed"*.

But, how do we tell the difference between lingering illness compensation (dysfunction) and healthy brain activity?

The thing to do (and it seems strangely simple) is ASK.

Yes, ask the patient, but especially, *especially* ask the patient's relatives! *That's the thing most chiropractors don't do.* They ask the patient a myriad of questions but ignore the second greatest source of information: the patient's relatives and close friends.

Patients are not always a reliable source when it comes to talking about themselves and their own health. They are too close to themselves to take notice of the bigger picture. **They are not seeing the forest for the trees!** But relatives are excellent gauges of a person's well-being. Not only are they likely more willing to talk or remember about certain past events (i.e. illnesses and injuries), but relatives will notice if someone is changing in their general mood, cognition, or speech.

And it's hard to know what questions to ask the patient themselves because, very simply put, one of the earliest signs and/or symptoms of brain dysfunction is memory loss. The patient might not be able to point to changes in their ability to remember what someone said, or they might think it's normal to have to write up shopping lists more frequently or make notes all over the place where they didn't before. They might simply attribute these changes to age, which is all wrong!

These are a certain signs that something is happening to the memory, in the brain.

Fatigue
Extreme tiredness usually as a result of mental or physical illness or exertion.

Like list-making and note-taking behaviours, people are not always aware of themselves and their habits, especially if they develop those habits over a period of time.

TIRED OF BEING TIRED

Another symptom of brain decline is fatigue. Fatigue experienced while working, driving, or learning (e.g. during a class) is a very, very important clue. If it exists, it's a certain sign that the brain is in trouble. *Always* **ask patients about fatigue.** The following questions provide a good base from which to start assessing a patient's level of fatigue:

- Do you tire easily when you are driving?
- Do you get unexplainably tired while at work?
- Do you feel like you need to take more naps, or like you've had to start napping?
- Is your capacity to learn and to retain information decreasing or is it improving?

FOCUS, DIGESTION, AND DRIVE

Loss of focus and concentration is another sign of brain dysfunction. Though short-term, high-stress situations can cause similar symptoms that disappear when the stress does, **when cortisol levels remain too high for too long a person can suffer from a more enduring loss of focus and concentration.** Whether from stress or not, loss of focus and concentration points to a decline in the brain, and that can spell big trouble for the body that you—the chiropractor—could easily recognise: poor posture, a decrease in spatial awareness, effects to autonomic functions like blood pressure, heart rate and rhythm, breathing, etc., and gut function.

Gastro-intestinal function is a special one. When there are problems with digestion and

---

"FACT" DEBUNK

Most people (even those who claim to know a lot about the brain and nervous system), have adopted the odd idea that the brain's functions are *supposed* to decline as we age.

This is absolutely NOT true!

Research has shown that people can maintain high brain function throughout their lives, if only they would work at it. We have to consistently challenge our brains. We have to keep learning, moving our bodies (providing basic stimulation and brain activity), and keep the brain activated as a whole.

elimination, almost surely it is a consequence of what is happening in the brain. So…

When it comes to function
OPTIMAL BRAIN = OPTIMAL GUT

Just think of all the mucus in the brain and the vast blood supply moving through brain tissue. The same goes with the motility of the gastro-intestinal tract: lots of mucus, lots of blood. You could say the brain is conversing with the gut via those blood and mucus tracts.

One of the earliest signs of brain decline in the elderly is a problem with the gastro-intestinal function, specifically constipation. The same applies to children with ADHD, especially children with Autism: they face the same gastro-intestinal problems as the elderly. *If that is the case then, surely, improper gut function can't all be due to age!*

(Other than gastro-intestinal function, ADHD/Autistic children often suffer auto-immune problems because the immune system is directly controlled by the brain. But that's outside of the contents of this report.)

A lack of drive or a change in motivation is another sure sign that the brain is going south. A lack of drive and motivation, of course, can be a short-lived because of immediate circumstances (e.g. you are unhappy with your job), but, whether short- or long-lived, the brain is calling for help. There are things that can be done to support the brain's function during difficult periods in life so that that situation doesn't result in lasting negative effects.

TOO MANY SIGNS TO LIST

There are a large number of other symptoms and signs which point to the possibility (nay, the likelihood!) that the brain is experiencing trouble. In fact, there are too many symptoms to continue listing out and describing them, each and every one, as I've done thus far.

Therefore, I've created a list of major symptoms I've already talked about as well as others I haven't to help you to quickly identify signs of brain dysfunction with your patients. You'll find it at the end of the chapter.

I encourage you to read over this list several times to get a good feel for what you should be looking for when interviewing and testing your patients. Once you become aware and identify any brain problems, follow up with a neurological and physical examination★ with specific focus on the motoric consequences of the brain.

I know this is a lot to take in. But, trust me.

It'll be undoubtedly difficult (especially if you've been practicing a while) to integrate these new processes into your routine. However, once you do it, *you'll begin changing the lives of your patients and for yourself in ways you would have never anticipated possible.* You'll receive a lot more reward with and in the work you do, and you'll be better able to understand *what* you are doing and pass along that understanding and trust to your patients.

Though I'm only giving you a short run-through in this report, you'll be able to use the steps I'm giving you as foundation to opening your mind and, ultimately, **mastering the relationship between the brain and the postural system.**

★*Though this chapter is entitled "Neurological Examination",* **it's important to also conduct a physical examination** *to make sure that the muscular tone in the spine and postural system has adapted or is adapting appropriately to changing circumstances.*

Signs of Brain Dysfunction

Poor posture	High/Low blood pressure
Decrease in spatial awareness	Slow Reflexes / Hypermobility
Fatigue	Decrease in memory and concentration
Digestive problems *(e.g. constipation, IBS)*	Lack of drive and/or changes in motivation
Learning difficulties *(e.g. slower than usual learning)*	Depression and/or anxiety
Changes in walking and general mobility	Changes in sense of smell
Changes in vital signs *(e.g. irregular heartbeat)*	Changes in muscle tone and coordination, and muscular imbalances
Hunched/slouched posture	Problems sleeping
Abnormal eye movement	Other mental and psychiatric problems
Decreased system oxygenation	Circulatory problems
Fluctuating (too high/too low) glucose levels	Chronic stress
Body pH (acidity)	Mood & personality changes
Spatial awareness problems	Poor nutrition
Frequent illness *(e.g. colds, migraines)*	Trouble balancing

Table 1

Examine patients for any of the listed signs and symptoms to determine if and what kind of brain dysfunction exists and, from there, determine what steps need to be taken in order to properly treat the problem(s).

CHAPTER 8

MAJOR & MINOR MOVEMENTS

One of the first things that change when the brain loses its grip on the postural system is the way you walk. Some of the bigger changes to take note of are:

- The arm-shoulder swing shortens *on the side of the brain's decline*;
- An in-rotation of the arms;
- A lesser amplitude of stride;
- A widened stance in order to remain more stable (just one of the ways the body compensates).

By doing something as easy as looking at how your patients move—how they walk, the speed with which they walk, the length of their stride, the stability that they have—you'll be able to tell if there's something going on that's a cause for greater concern.

Other than walking, take a look at their vitals. For instance, look for changes in blood pressure or in how they breathe. Do they breathe shallow or deeply? Has there been a change in their heart rhythm and rate?

Look at posture and at the gait. Has the patient adopted a slump in their shoulders, a hunch in their back, or an in-rotation of the shoulders? What about the head itself: is there forward or backward carriage of the head? And the face: do you see eye white above or under the eyes (pupils)?

(Remember Mary and how her seemingly unassociated symptoms—change in gait, pace, concentration, stance—were all caused by brain dysfunction?)

Any postural or spatial awareness changes are signs that something is happening in the brain. The body will adapt to changes in the brain by changing posture and, thus, adopt all the consequences that go with it: pain, headaches, numbness, fatigue between the shoulder blades, neck problems, shoulder problems, and problems in the lower back.

CHIROPRACTORS ARE ALL TOO FAMILIAR WITH TREATING THESE *SYMPTOMS*, BUT **WE RARELY TREAT THE UNDERLYING CAUSE.**

Often we—not just chiropractors, but people in general—tend to think that postural changes are due to spinal dysfunction or a lack of nutritional supplementations, or spinal injuries. *But, in reality, posture changes are often due to a changing brain.* And the brain can and needs to be treated to bring it back to a healthy state.

Granted, there are people out there who suffer spinal injuries and spinal dysfunction *whose posture doesn't change.* Why is this? It's because, either consciously or not, they're aware of the brain-postural relationship and they're keeping their brains healthy as a part of their healthcare regimen. And even if they shrink a little bit in muscle mass because they can't exercise the way they used to (muscular atrophy), or they get older, or are physically handicapped because of an injury, they do not lose the majesty of a "young" posture.

A healthy brain will show outwardly in a posture which looks like the following:

...strong pose, shoulders rolled back...

...a good, firm stance, equally balanced...

...head upright, not held forward or backward...

...feet very close together while walking...

...and kept close together when standing.

Postural balance is one of the first things that will go wrong when the brain goes south.

In the typical chiropractic patient the posture goes awry first, but we normally attribute it to not enough muscle strength [in the shoulders and upper back] or poor posture. We then suggest the patient do some muscle strengthening exercise or simply remind them to sit up. But those solutions don't work. Why not? Because if the source of the problem is in the brain, doing minor strength training or simply remembering to sit up straight won't fix it!

It's a devious circle of influence—the brain to posture, and posture to brain—that traditional chiropractics have failed to fix at the source. Instead, the weed is clipped at the leaf while the root continues to grow.

Alongside posture is spatial awareness. I don't know many chiropractors who take a careful look at spatial awareness and balance in an initial consultation or even in a follow-up appointment. Perhaps they do in passing, or if there is a very obvious problem that simply can't be overlooked or if the patient brings up the topic directly. But spatial awareness isn't tested as a strict part of their assessment. So, now I ask...

DO YOU ACTIVELY ASSESS
SPATIAL AWARENESS AND BALANCE?

If not, it's time to bring your patient's healthcare file and history up to speed.

Do a Romberg's test on a foam cushion and see if your patient is able to correct themselves actively and without problems. Have them stand on each leg individually and see how long they can hold themselves there without falling over.

One of the easiest things you can do to see if a patient's brain is still functioning at the rate it should be is to test their capacity to defeat gravity, to stand upright and properly, *not* slumping forward.

We take standing up for granted because it's normal for human beings to do so. If it's so easy, then why do we awe at a gorilla that regularly walks like a man? Or at a dog that can stand up and walk on its hind legs?

DOCTOR'S NOTE
We're all different. We all have different norms.
As with all medically-related tests, it's important to do
them at regular intervals so you have an idea of where
the baseline for that individual person is. I strongly
encourage you to start monitoring postural traits with
all your patients and make good, detailed notes of how
they tested so that you can compare from visit to visit
what's happening with that patient over time.

Standing Up: More than It Seems

Revert back to when I mentioned the chiropractor and the visual
practice and that it's what makes us different and more aptly
positioned among other healthcare professionals to treat brain
dysfunction. Alongside that, remember that I said it isn't only the
postural muscles that work to keep us standing up: it's our entire
system. More specifically, the Area Acoustica of the brain and the
deep spinal muscles working in tandem.

Postural muscle control, deep spinal muscles, eye muscles, and
the coordination of all of these... That's a lot of work the brain is
putting in just to keep us standing upright! So when our brain starts
losing capacity to handle such a huge task, we *chiropractors* will easily
notice those signs outwardly.

*The vestibular system is one of the systems that we as chiropractors should
master because this system is most directly related to the spine.* It's the system
that keeps the spine upright, keeps the body upright, and provides spatial
orientations together with the higher hemispheric control centres.

WHEN OUR BRAIN STARTS
LOSING ITS CAPACITY TO
HANDLE STANDING,
**WE CHIROPRACTORS
WILL SEE THE SIGNS.**

Balance is a beautiful, fluid thing. Our bodies are programmed so that if one part fails a little bit, your body naturally and automatically compensates with another part. The information gathered from vision, from the spinal muscles, from hearing (inner ears), all combine as minute and infinite signals sent to the brain and all work together to keep us upright and perfectly balanced.

But the reality is less beautiful: in almost all of us, one of these systems is not working properly (dysfunctional). While this imbalance usually isn't a problem because our bodies compensate, there are some people whose imbalances cause a lot of harm either immediately or down the road.

If a patient experienced head trauma when they were young— where they were knocked unconscious, had to receive stitches in their head, were in a car accident—as they start to get older their so-thought "healed" injury will resurface as, perhaps, a sudden spell of dizziness or difficulty standing without help from a cane to help them balance. **While to the regular eye these problems may seem new, they aren't**: they were existing issues stemming from childhood in what we call the central vestibular integration at brain level.

And this vestibular system, as I have said before, has a great influence on the spinal balance and on the spatial awareness of your body. And if that goes wrong your body will suddenly start to adjust, to make compensations through unnatural (though discreet) movements in the spine and postural system.

Compensations which lead to spinal problems and pain.

So, looking at it this way, it's obvious that you don't just want to address the spine or the shoulders or the legs or the hips as traditional chiropractics would suggest. *Now we know we need to also look at what's happening in the brain.* As a doctor, you need to:

increase the brain's ability to compensate
and
decrease these imbalances through chiropractic treatment.

Testing balance is simple: have your patient stand on one leg for a few seconds, and then the other. If your patient sways more on one side than the other side, or has more difficulty on one side than the other, *that's abnormal.* Balance, as its name implies, should be equal.

A Fukuda's Test is another great way to determine brain-body imbalances. (It's also called an Fukuda Stepping Test or Unterberger Step Test.) With the eyes closed and both hands held out in front, have your patient start marching in place. If they start leaning into one side a little bit more, there's a bigger problem at hand.

ALL SEEING EYES

Now we understand that we have a visual practice taking view of the body as a whole. The Area Acoustica works to keep us upright and our observations as skilled chiropractors are working to resolve problems (i.e. pain) from unnatural movements in the postural system and the deep spinal muscles caused by compensations.

One step further again:

> The deep spinal muscles are directly related to the
> **eye muscles and the control of the eye muscles.**

So how important are the eye muscles in assessing brain problems?
Critically so.
Because the eyes are not just the window to the soul: they're the window to the brain. The eyes are one of the few mechanisms in the body that are related to ALL other parts of the nervous system—not the back, not the arms, not even the head, but the *eyes.*
Looking at the eyes, at the eyes' movements, will give you great insight as to what's happening in the brain.
We're not optometrists or ophthalmologists, but we can do a basic eye examination from the comfort of our own office without the use of specialized equipment, intimidating procedures, or long processes. And, by "basic examination," I mean looking to see that the eye muscles are functioning the way they should be.
What precisely are we looking for? Well, let's first start with a quick process:
Tell your patient to look at a specific target (e.g. the tip of a pen or the tip of your finger), and to follow that target with their

eyes as you move it left-right-up-down-diagonally. Then hold the target off to one side and then the other for a few seconds at a time, forcing your patient to hold a sideways gaze without moving the head (but be careful not to go beyond the eyes' natural range of motion, as that is rather unfair). While you do this, **closely observe the patient's eye movements together, and then individually, left and right.** See what is happening and go through this simple checklist:

- **Are the eyes moving in a regular way: smoothly and with little effort?**
- **Are there pursuits or saccades?** (Pursuits are fluid following motions, while saccades are jumping movements from one space to another.)
- **Is it difficult for the patient to hold a gaze to one side or another?**
- **Is there a difference in eye muscle movement from one side to another?**

What you want to see are smooth, easy eye movements while pursuing a target; there shouldn't be any jolting or jumping as the eyes follow the designated object around. As with balance, BOTH sides should function this way. *If there are differences between them, there's something wrong.*

As you can see, both of these tests are about subtlety. Truly, all these tests for brain trouble are.

MAKING OLFACTORY SENSE

Another big clue that the brain is beginning to deteriorate is that the patient will start having olfactory problems. Again understand that your patients may not tell you they're having problems with smell… in fact, they may not even KNOW they have problems with smell! So, once again, you need to test it.

If you're just out of chiropractic school you're probably more likely to test smell than those of us who have been practicing for a while. **If you're anything like me, you'll just forget about doing it.** I can bet that the typical chiropractor will not routinely assess smell after the first year of practice. But we all should, because a loss of olfactory sense is one of the early indicators of a neurological disease or brain dysfunction.

(Because conducting olfactory testing is likely something we all learned to do while in school, I won't bother to explain a procedure here.)

HISTORICALLY SPEAKING

I believe chiropractors differ from all the other healthcare professions that deal with problems in the postural system because we are very good at asking for a patient's trauma history. Sure, allopathic doctors might ask about one's *healthcare* history, but, for many patients, a healthcare history is not inclusive of incidents specific to trauma or injury.

And we chiropractors know that trauma is where the problems start.

Not only are we concerned about medicinal history as it relates to conditions, genetics, medications/prescriptions, and surgeries, but we'll more commonly ask our patients two basic questions:

"HAVE YOU HAD ANY CHILDHOOD TRAUMA?"
"HAVE YOU BEEN IN ANY CAR ACCIDENTS?"

Traditionally, chiropractors have asked these questions to determine if there are any injuries to the tendons, muscles, or joints; scarring or tissues from an improper heal. Basically, we're looking for injuries to the postural system.

However, we shouldn't only be concerned about scars and whiplash.

We need to know about past trauma in order to help us detect compensations in the brain at the vestibular level. While the healthcare community as a whole will admit there's a direct relation between knocks in the head and an *immediate* increase in the likelihood of brain problems (e.g. swelling, bleeding), little does anyone take into consideration the long-term and distant effects of head injury.

The blood brain barrier opens up like a released dam after a good blow on the head. Neural inflammation follows this release, and can proceed for years and years and years. **If you have a patient who has experienced severe trauma to the head, you need to do something to decrease these inflammatory processes,** *even if the trauma occurred some time ago.*

Furthermore, if you improve overall brain health, you will improve the brain's capacity to decrease its inflammatory reaction. And that's a huge relief, because

IMPROVING THE BRAIN'S CAPACITY TO HEAL ITSELF
IS MUCH EASIER THAN TRYING TO
CONTROL THE INFLAMMATION DIRECTLY.

For example, you can suggest (or prescribe) to the patient a botanical supplement like curcumin (a main component in the spice turmeric), Resveratrol (a natural phenol found in grape skins, peanuts [sprouted], mulberry, and dark chocolate), and/or magnesium to decrease the effects of these brain traumas.

OVERVIEW

The main mantra of this and the previous chapter is to BE AWARE. **Be aware that there may be problems lurking behind unlikely symptoms.** Do a proper and thorough examination. Look at the motoric consequences which are under control of the brain, not just at the arm and leg movements but all of the movements, down to the movements of the eyes.

And, while motorics are important, that's only a small part of the bigger assessment.

Look at autonomic function. For example, differences in blood pressure could be a reflection of differences in hemispheric function.

Look at the ability to stand upright, to move the eyes, how the olfactory sense is operating. Look for differences in tonicity of the muscles. And look at the fatigue-ability from one side to another.

These are all indications that something may be wrong with the brain.

CHAPTER 9

TREATMENT & SUPPORTIVE CONSIDERATIONS

Toward the end of the last chapter I read off a short list of supplements an individual could take to assist with reducing inflammation in the brain.

That's only the beginning of the fun.

What I'm going to share with you now in regard to treatment considerations are just the fundamentals for how the brain can and *should* function, and some suggestions as to how to help it out if you notice it's headed for (or is already in) trouble.

BACK TO THE BASICS (AGAIN)

Once more, let's remind ourselves of that list of three things the brain requires to properly function:

ASSUMPTION crush

Remember that this report deals primarily with *raising your awareness.*

While I'm happy to share some ways I help to improve the brain health of my own patients', it's ultimately up to you to delve into the deeper studies and read publications that explain the types of supplementations and benefits thereof available to both the physician and the everyday consumer (and, trust me, there are plenty! For starters, take a look at my own list of **references**.).

OXYGEN

NUTRITION

ENVIRONMENTAL STIMULATION

There you go again. The three things you need to give your brain in order to help it function at its optimal level. And the brain is a great pal: in return, it works hard to keep *you* alive, to help *you* function optimally.

It's a simple and effective tit-for-tat.

As the body evolves from childhood to adulthood it becomes more and more capable of providing for your brain's needs in a more gracious way. Your blood pressure stabilizes. Your heart rate stabilizes. (Nutrition comes through nutrients in the blood stream.) Your breathing deepens, steadies, becomes more stable. (Oxygen also travels through the blood stream.) And, when you exercise (i.e. stimulate), these stabilize even more.

Ergo: oxygen, nutrition, stimulation.

But it's apparent that even the adult brains of the world aren't in their best shape.

When there's indication that the brain may be in trouble, that's where you need to start looking: oxygen, nutrition, and stimulation. Those are the only three points you need to address in conjunction with (NOT "*in lieu of*"!) your standard chiropractic treatment.

START WITH AIR

It's no mistake that "oxygen" is at the top of our three-piece list. Seeing that the brain is being sufficiently oxygenated should be your very first step in aiding it in recovery.

When it comes to oxygenation, EMS (Emergency Medical Services) and first aid professionals know their ABC's: airway, breathing, circulation. Those three key words assist in improving breathing during any number of urgent situations. However, the ABC's aren't only for emergencies, but could help us in the long run, too.

DOCTOR'S NOTE

We're all different. And so are our brains.

Though I'm the last person to tell you what to do with your patients — how to treat them, what to treat them for — I ask that you remember to adapt your methods to the individual being treated. The worst thing you can do for your patients and your practice is to adopt a generic, cover-all protocol when you sense something is wrong in the brain. Different underlying problems require different medical approaches.

Some brains may not be able to handle a treatment as well as another; likewise, a successful treatment in one does not equal success in another. A patient might seem to be handling a treatment well, but it's up to *you* to determine if that is true. After all, they didn't know anything was wrong in the first place! How could they tell you it's all right now? Monitor progress carefully while remembering it's easy to get overzealous with treatments.

We want to improve oxygen flow in the body. Your brain depends on it.

Here are suggestions as to how you might do that:

Make spinal adjustments accordingly. Our standard practice tells us *to improve breathing we need to improve spinal mobility and appropriate spinal curves.* A lordotic and mobile lumbar spine will help the diaphragm to completely lower so that the lungs can completely fill.

Teach for long-term benefit. As I did for Mary, it's possible to make postural changes to open the airways and optimize ventilation. Of course, use treatment techniques to improve breathing and to improve blood flow to and from the lungs in a more immediate manner, but you can also influence the airways by, for example, teaching your patient how to perform a Brugger's relief position or educating them in techniques of deep abdominal breathing.

Let's give an example of how this kind of treatment might go:

Imagine you have a low back patient with a decrease in lumbar curvature. They're likely experiencing stiffness, pain, and paraspinal spasms; their posture is likely slumped and the diaphragm is being restricted. *Using traditional chiropractic methods will address these pain issues, certainly, but they're also going to help improve the patient's breathing.*

We know from experience that improving spinal mobility and curvature will assist in lowering the diaphragm. Lowered diaphragm equals better breathing.

Great! You've both nixed the pain and improved breathing. You're done, right?

Nope. Not if you want to keep it from happening again. Because, remember: traditional chiropractic techniques merely fix symptoms, *not the root cause*, which is the BRAIN.

Now is the time to go above and beyond your patient's expectations.

Let's say that, on top of the traditional treatment, you show your patient some breathing exercises, perhaps give them a flyer with instructions for Brugger's. You show them how they should control their posture, how they should hold their head and pull back their shoulders, maybe even how they can exercise the shoulder muscles to help keep the shoulders from slumping forward.

Not only will you greatly improve the base activation of the brain by improving spinal activation [through standard treatment], but you'll also be improving breathing and oxygenation of *all* the tissues including the most important ones: those in the brain.

You've addressed airways and breathing, the patient feels better, and that's great, but those are only the first two steps in our ABC's of oxygenation.

The last is circulation.

> BY GOING BEYOND
> EXPECTATION, YOU'LL
> **IMPROVE ALL THE**
> **TISSUES OF THE BODY,**
> INCLUDING THOSE IN THE
> **BRAIN.**

Circulation is special in that it addresses two of the three components for optimal brain health: oxygen and nutrition. The easiest thing to do when trying to improve circulation is to monitor your patient's blood pressure. *If blood pressure is too high or too low that means circulation is compromised: less oxygen is getting to the brain and fewer nutrients are getting to the brain, too.* There are supplements and botanicals—like fish oil, ginseng, B vitamins, hibiscus, or garlic—that have an influence over blood pressure so it regulates to an appropriate level.

WARNING
If a patient's blood pressure is **dangerously high or low**, sending them straight to their family physician for **an acute intervention** instead of treating with supplements and botanicals may be the right choice.

Blood pressure is a funny thing and affects us in ways we wouldn't even realise. If you take a careful look at your patient population there are likely cases of patients who have experienced a long period of untraceable problems. **Once their blood pressure becomes regulated, either by pharmaceutical medication or in a more holistic way, and the problems seem to dissipate.** That's just one example of how the brain is able to regain control over posture and pain.

SUGAR, SUGAR!

Though we need a certain amount of sugar in our bodies to thrive, most people indulge too heartily in foods that both contain and convert to sugar: sweets, syrups, carbohydrates, and alcohol.

Regulating glucose levels is crucial for a healthy brain.
You may have heard about something called The Cavemen Diet.
Essentially, it's taking away the carbohydrates and thereby helping to
regulate the body's glucose levels. Magnesium as a supplement and in
high-content foods such as black beans, pumpkin seeds, and spinach,
works to protect the brain from the damaging effects of too much
glucose, and also helps regulate glucose levels at the cellular level.

Also, eating more frequently and in lesser portions will assist in
avoiding sugar "highs" and the unavoidable "crashes". Eating the
largest meals in the morning and tapering off to the smallest meals
in the evening will also help, as there's no sense in gorging in the
evening if that food energy isn't going to be used productively (to
work, play, or through other activity). Likely, a too-full tummy
before bed will also result in either a less beneficial sleep as the sugars
from the food try to burn off, or into a conversion into fat as the
body makes efforts to store the energy for another day. (If, however,
someone has low glucose levels at night, eating a small snack before
bedtime can aid the brain's performance throughout the night and
immediately upon waking.)

*Most importantly, glucose directly competes with the performance of your
brain's neurotransmitters,* so you absolutely want to monitor glucose
levels for optimal brain health. Too much glucose will also make the
brain oversensitive to input and information, which is why sugar-
stimulated children (and adults!) find it hard to concentrate.

A BODILY PH-ACT

While the body's glucose level is most often thought to be the only
drawback of ingesting sugars, that's not the only damage sugars do.
When sugars are digested and ingested, they also decrease the body's
pH and increase the acidity.

The fact is that most people's bodies are too acidic.

The body functions best in a slightly alkaline state, so having a
too-acid pH (a pH *below* 7.4 is considered acidic for the human body)
can wreak havoc on both the body and the brain. People nowadays
eat foods that are high in carbohydrates, sugars, and red proteins
(foods that up the acidity) and take in too few green vegetables,
which alkalize the body. Alongside food, their beverage choices are all

wrong! *People who suffer from a too-acidic pH generally don't drink enough water.* Instead they opt for sugar-packed and acid-producing beverages: coffee, tea, juices, lemonade, alcohol, or sodas.

Optimising the body's pH will immensely assist the brain in governing and monitoring your body's other vital functions.

Improving your patient's diet to include more green vegetables and fewer sugars won't only help to regulate glucose and pH, but will also help decrease inflammatory reactions in the body. *This includes* brain *inflammation!* Whenever there has been brain trauma and you feel there might be a lingering chronic brain inflammation, you want your patient to change their diet. Get them to take away the carbohydrates, and eat more green vegetables, lean meat, and fish.

IMMUNITY MALFUNCTION

Consider the immune system and ask your patient the following questions:

- Do you get sick easily, or often?
- Do you have any signs of chronic allergic reaction *that you know of* (e.g. inflammation, brain fog, fatigue, headache)?
- Are there substances *that you know of* that you have a reaction to?
- Do you have any allergies *that you know of?*

"FACT" DEBUNK

There are organisations which praise the safety of agricultural pesticides. But, science takes time, so... how could they really know?

Chemical pesticides are still relatively new to humankind's food growing process.

Chemical pesticides only began to be regularly used in food production in the 1950s. So, no matter what anybody says, we simply and scientifically do not know with certainty what the chemicals sprayed onto our foods do to our *long-term health.*

There just hasn't been enough time to tell.

In my experience with many children who are diagnosed with ADHD/Autism, I've found that they are likelier to have so-called delayed immune reactions next to the more obvious immediate and acute ones. Many children benefit from abstaining from certain foods. *Many parents of my ADHD/Autism patients find that their children's problems sprang from a list of food allergies they didn't know they had!*

In knowing that, it may well be that there are some food substances or substances in your patient's environment that are causing adverse allergic reactions. And notice I italicised "that you know of" in the above-listed questions. That's important because, again, I'll say: **your patient does not always *know* when they are sick!** What a patient may deem as a "regular" headache or "normal" brain fogginess today may be due to the milk product they ate 1-2 days ago, or that cleaning agent they were exposed to yesterday.

So, to sum up, we've gone over...

...the first ingredient for an optimally functioning brain—oxygenation—and its related ABC's (airway, breathing, circulation)...

...how circulation is both oxygenation *and* nutrition (the second brain ingredient)...

...how you can help your patient to support their brain nutritionally, not just with a change in diet (e.g. omitting sugars, more green vegetables) but also by looking at nutritional choices in a different way (e.g. how foods affect the body's pH and the adverse effects of "hidden" allergies).

But, even if your patient changes to a healthier lifestyle, you may still want to give them some additional support.

NUTRITIONAL CONSIDERATIONS

This section focuses on recommendations and various considerations—treatments, supplements—on how to improve your patient population's brain health. Some of these are well-researched and widely used, while others have just recently been publicised as being helpful for the brain.

I do not intend to continue on without addressing our third factor for optimal brain health—environmental stimulation—and how it directly connects to nutrition.

I'll address that now.

It's no surprise that most people do not regularly stimulate their minds or muscles. Life, for many, fails to challenge us in ways that will keep our brains sharp and active, or our muscles and reflexes in good shape.

I believe a lifestyle change—one in which a person challenges their cognitive and emotional abilities and challenges their body to move—in your patient population is one of the best ways to promote good brain health.

But, even if all your patients did this, you could still help them achieve more through nutritional supplementation.

It's rare for a person to obtain all the necessary nutrients the body (and brain) need through diet alone. For those who do, they are probably the lucky few who will never experience brain dysfunction in their lifetime.

Let's consider Mary yet again: her condition improved and pelvic pains disappeared by changing her diet, taking supplements, and doing some basic brain exercises.

Note I did NOT say *muscular* exercises.

While the brain exercises were critical to Mary's recovery, the supplements I encouraged her to take were also vital to her brain having the "fuel" it needed to be able to perform in a capacity to *do* those exercises. In other words, without the nutrients, no manner of mental exercises would be fruitful. (The one I specifically mentioned in Chapter 4 were Omega 3s high in DHA.)

Omega 3s are, essentially, your fish oils. But—beware!—not all fish oils are made equal! In fact, most fish oils are ill-suited for optimising brain health. Be sure your patients seek out oil supplementations *high in DHA,* not the EPA that most of them contain. Omega 3, krill, and cod liver oils are all examples of fish oils high in DHA.

Another brain nutritive is a supplement becoming more and more popular, especially as people spend more and more time indoors and less time outside. **I'm talking about Vitamin D-3, also known as the "sunshine vitamin",** which can be obtained from some foods but is mostly manufactured by the body when exposed to sunlight. Research shows that a high proportion of people in the Nordic hemisphere and in the modern western countries have a deficiency in Vitamin D-3.

Vitamin D-3 not only makes sure certain neurotransmitters [brain chemicals] are produced, thereby stimulating brain performance, but a lack of it can result in *brain dysfunction* in addition to:

...muscle weakness...

...bone pain...

...depression...

...and an increased risk for Type 2 Diabetes.

Vitamin D-3 is a great immune system supporter—people who are D-3 deficient will experience more illnesses, flues, and colds than those who ingest adequate amounts of D-3. *Besides this, D-3 is considered one of the most potent immune regulators.* Taking a high dose of Vitamin D can actually be of great benefit when suffering from an autoimmune condition (e.g. Rheumatoid arthrosis, Hashimoto's thyroid disease). While I encourage all individuals to take a D-3 supplement (because a high dosage or "overdose" of D-3 will not harm you), **I especially encourage those with auto-immune diseases or disorders to take VERY high doses.**

DOCTOR'S NOTE
Picking for your Brain.
If you ever go out into the fields or woods for a hike or picnic, don't pass up an opportunity to do your brain some good when you spot a few morsels on a nearby bush or vine. <u>Bilberries and other fruits of the forest are jam-packed with brain nutrients.</u> Most potent if picked wild, they contain antioxidants, a plethora of vitamins, and other specific substances (e.g. amino acids, trace minerals and substances such as anthocianins) which are strongly neuroprotective.

To B, or Not to B

B vitamins play a critical role in brain health and the general public is finally catching on. Products are coming out on the market advertising high B vitamin content, B Vitamin complexes, and their relation to mental acuity and bodily (and mental) energy.

B-12, B-6, and pantothenic acid (also known as pantothenate or B-5) all play a very important role in memory.

Acety-who? The Little Compound that Could

Acetylcholine: a little compound in your temporal cortex that helps with memory, cognition, and is claimed to even raise intelligence levels!

As the brain's most common neurotransmitter, acetylcholine could use a little help with all the work it does.

When people start to show a decline in their brain functions, usually in regard to memory, spatial orientation, and reading skills, then there's no doubt that acetylcholine levels have been affected.

And, while science hasn't found a way to create a "pure" form of directly ingestible acetylcholine, taking supplements such as a B Vitamin Complex, Ginko Biloba, Alpha GPC, Bacopa Monnieri, and/or DMAE can help your patient's brain metabolize, maintain, mimic, or produce more acetylcholine.

Supplementation is something that will make a very big difference in some patients. *But, never forget that you can never just give a supplement!* Supplements are often prescribed by healthcare professionals as "fix all" solutions when they're really only one of the many components of the brain's first aid kit. It takes the entire package to really improve your patient's health: exercise, stimulation, nutrition, stress management, et cetera.

Never forget to ask yourself:

- What do my patients eat?
- How much do they move?
- How much do they stimulate themselves mentally and physically?

- Do they do things to reduce their stress levels?

Looking at Mary's efforts individually is good for analyses sake, but let's step back for a moment to move away from the trees and see the whole forest:

In the broader picture, what Mary did was make a lifestyle change that changed her life.

CHAPTER 10

LIFESTYLE CHANGES

Hands down, for most people it's important to conduct a lifestyle intervention. Saying "intervention" may appear overtly serious, but it really is that important. This is your patient's *brain* on the line, after all! Unlike other vital organs (e.g. heart, skin, liver, kidneys, lungs) which can be repaired, or sometimes even replaced, by surgical methods, there is no such thing as a "brain transplant". We have ONE chance to take care of our brains, and we need to seriously consider the consequences of not doing just that.

To tell patients to "change your lifestyle" is very simplistic. Certainly there are any number of things to do, habits to break, views to modify... and those are no easy tasks.

> WE HAVE
> **ONE CHANCE TO TAKE**
> **CAREOF OUR BRAINS,**
> AND WE NEED TO
> SERIOUSLY CONSIDER
> **THE CONSEQUENCES OF**
> **NOT DOING JUST THAT.**

But, let's start with that simplified view, that single phrase—"change your lifestyle"—if only to get us pointed in the right direction.

CHANGE BEGINS WITH MOTION

It's not enough to merely say, "Change, or else such-and-such will happen." **People are believers in physical action; as a species, we tend to believe with our eyes rather than with our minds or hearts.** And your patients are no different: they'll want to *feel* and *see* that things are happening.

For instance, though there are benefits to exercises that don't cause muscular soreness the next day, most people aren't convinced that their efforts did anything because they can't *feel* the results in their bodies. Examples of those kinds of exercises might be simple stretching routines that don't cause soreness but will, over time, improve flexibility, or doing only a few push-ups each night that aren't enough to cause soreness, but will improve arm, shoulder, and core strength as the practice continues.

So, instead of merely saying, "Change your lifestyle," tell them instead, "Move your brain."

If they give you a questioning stare, add this in:

Literally. Start using your body.

The human system improves itself with motion. If you are not moving, which most of us do not do enough of, you will deteriorate. Your muscles deteriorate, your organs deteriorate, your brain deteriorates. **Moving is very important for your whole body, *especially* for your brain.**

The brain is hardwired with your movement system. And I do mean "movement system", not exclusively the musculatory system. Not just muscles need moving, but tendons, ligaments, the movement of blood throughout the body (circulation), the motion of the lungs as they expand and contract and the resulting airflow (respiration)… *everything in your body that moves effects the function of the brain.*

Let me say it again:

If you don't move, your brain *WILL* deteriorate.

Look at the graphic on the following page to see how you might suggest to your patients they start moving their brains.

Take on new challenges.

- Learn a new language.

-Learn a new skill.

-Meet new people.

-Adopt a pet.

- Join a social club or sports league.

Do new things, or do old things in a new way.

Take a different route to work, or try carpooling to add some spice to a dull commute.

Change routines, or break them altogether.

- Do the same activities at different times of day (e.g. jogging at night instead of morning)

Expand your current knowledge of a favourite activity or topic.

- If you road bike, try mountain biking, or vice versa.

Graphic 1
Examples of activities which will help keep the brain in motion.

MAINTAIN BALANCE: SLEEP & STRESS

Alongside moving, the brain also needs its downtime. If your patient is experiencing sleep issues, don't waive them off as "normal" because "everyone has to deal with sleep problems"... that is, from 17-20% of the population.[2]

Address your patient's sleep issues directly and with fervour.

Why?

Because sleep is one of the body's most important mechanisms for keeping your brain in tip-top shape. Not getting enough sleep means your brain isn't getting its chance to absorb the new things it's learned and heal itself.

And I'm all about helping the brain heal itself.

And, if sleep is being compromised, there's a high likelihood that stress is a culprit.

Ask your patients sleep- and stress-specific questions, like...

- *Do you sleep soundly?*
- *Do you sleep enough (6-8 hours a night)?*
- *Do you have to regularly rely on a pharmaceutical (e.g. OTC Nytol) or depressant (e.g. an alcoholic "night cap") to fall and stay asleep?*
- *Do you experience anxiety (does your mind race) which prevents you from falling asleep?*
- *Do you wake up in the middle of the night then can't return to sleep?*
- *Have you ever been tested for, diagnosed with, or regularly experienced insomnia, sleep walking, sleep apnea, or another sleeping disorder?*

Though achieving six to eight hours of solid sleep a night (and that means *actual* sleeping, not just lying in bed) is a goal, we must remember: all things in moderation. More sleep isn't necessarily

---

2 According to a study done by the UK's University of Warwick Medical School, nearly 17% of the population in developing nations and nearly 20% of the population in developed nations experience sleep difficulties. http://www.psychologytoday.com/blog/sleep-newzzz/201208/are-sleep-problems-the-next-global-health-crisis.

better. *If a patient is sleeping excessively it's very indicative that something is wrong in the brain.* Too much sleep needs to be addressed just as seriously as not enough sleep.

Moving beyond addressing the problem(s), how do you go about helping your patient overcome their issue?

There are many ways to achieve better sleep for the body and the brain. It's possible to assist the body's natural inclination to fall asleep by taking a melatonin supplement or by drinking chamomile tea, which works as a mild tranquilizer and sleep inducer. Don't watch television for at least two hours before bedtime and try to avoid very intense emotional activities an hour before trying to sleep.

For a lot of people, a lack of sleep (or even an excess of sleep) is due to poor stress management practices. Too many people avoid addressing the stressful situation and just try to "sleep it off". *Stress needs to be actively managed: be aware that you have it, acknowledge it, then learn to put it aside.*

Exercising will help reduce stress and, thereby, improve sleep. And it doesn't have to be strenuous: taking a few minutes to stretch the tension out of muscles or a session of deep abdominal breathing or yoga should do the trick.

To battle anxiety, you can suggest starting a meditation regimen, either before bed to set aside the worries of the day or in the morning to prep the mind for the oncoming day. In addition to meditation, mindfulness is an excellent practice. There's much research that really points to the beneficial effects of meditation and mindfulness for both body and brain.

CHAPTER 11

FINDING THE MOTIVATION

Suggestions are great and your patient may seem happy, even eager, to comply when they're in the limelight of your examination room. As they sit listening to your advice, they're feeling encouraged: your insistence rubs off on them as a general's bravery rubs off on his soldiers in the midst of battle. But, once the battlefield is vacated in favour of familiar surroundings, the soldier quickly loses his resolve.

Humans are creatures of habit, and it's common for a person to shrug off changing to their new doctor-prescribed lifestyle in favour of routine.

And that's really discouraging for healthcare practitioners like us who are genuinely trying to help.

> ONCE THE BATTLEFIELD IS
> VACATED IN FAVOR OF
> FAMILIAR SURROUNDINGS,
> **THE SOLDIER QUICKLY
> LOSES HIS RESOLVE.**

Telling your patient their brain may be sick is hard. Asking them to make changes can be difficult. And having to face the disappointment of them not following your suggestions and watching their health deteriorate further can be heartbreaking.

So, how do you maintain your own motivation?

While I'd love to give you great words of advice in this area, I can't, other than to say it'll do wonders for you and your practice, and your patients (if they listen). **Like individualizing treatments for individual brains, there's no one answer.** It's a question only you can answer for yourself.

Still, by now I hope you've come to realise the truth behind brain health and how it affects our individual practices, the realm medicine of chiropractics, and, ultimately, the health of the world's population. I can only hope that that truth acts as a driving force, spurring you on.

I hope you'll remember the importance of oxygen, nutrition, and stimulation.

Above the rest, I hope you're able to maintain your motivation for learning about the brain after you put down this report. I can only wish that reading this report has hit some kind of chord with you; that from here on you'll begin looking *away from muscles and bones* and, instead, look at your patient's brain to see what influence it may be having on his or her condition; that you'll see how seemingly simple issues like a pulled muscle or an SI problem can stem from dysfunction in the brain.

The brain's capacity to control and to regulate the postural system, spine, and pain system is truly mindboggling.

Start asking questions. Create a simple questionnaire from what you've learned from this report (or use the one I've made). Do a proper examination... a COMPLETE examination. It may sound daunting, but takes less than three minutes to examine simple things like balance, eye movement, smell, and gait.

Make a note every time you examine, even if the note says "No changes". When you start noticing something different, write it down. **You never know when a seemingly insignificant detail will become a critical piece of information!**

And I know sometimes you may feel like you don't have the extra time. Even after all my experiences and all my knowledge, after dealing with my mother's situation and after working for so long with mentally disabled children, I still fell into the trap of feeling rushed and didn't listen to Mary when she came to see me the first time.

But if you at least try to be aware—to be mindful—you'll start developing a gut feeling for those small and critical symptoms of brain dysfunction.

As a refresher, here's that table listing those things to keep an open eye for during patient examination:

Signs of Brain Dysfunction	
Poor posture	High/Low blood pressure
Decrease in spatial awareness	Slow Reflexes / Hypermobility
Fatigue	Decrease in memory and concentration
Digestive problems (*e.g. constipation, IBS*)	Lack of drive and/or changes in motivation
Learning difficulties (*e.g. slower than usual learning*)	Depression and/or anxiety
Changes in walking and general mobility	Changes in sense of smell
Changes in vital signs (*e.g. irregular heartbeat*)	Changes in muscle tone and coordination, and muscular imbalances
Hunched/slouched posture	Problems sleeping
Abnormal eye movement	Other mental and psychiatric problems
Decreased system oxygenation	Circulatory problems
Fluctuating (too high/too low) glucose levels	Chronic stress
Body pH (acidity)	Mood & personality changes
Spatial awareness problems	Poor nutrition
Frequent illness (*e.g. colds, migraines*)	Trouble balancing

And, to help your patient's brain recover itself (because, again, it's easier to help the brain repair itself than to directly repair the brain!), I hope you'll strongly suggest they make changes to lifestyle habits and nutritional practices.

(And with the supplements, just like vitamins and minerals, you always want to make sure your patient reacts favourably to them: that no allergies are present, that the patient isn't experiencing adverse reactions or a lack of reaction at all. After all, you wouldn't want to keep pushing and wasting time with D-3 when it's not having an effect, or prescribing Omega 3s to someone with a fish allergy!)

As you practice doing examinations and taking notes, you'll become more attuned to observing what's going on.

It only takes one step to change *everything:* your practice, your patients' lives, and your own life.

So make that first step.

And don't do it out of obligation or automation. You have to take a sane, scientific, responsible, and reasonable approach to these individualistic problems your patients are experiencing when trying to use their brains.

In other words: you have to start using *your* brain as well.

CHAPTER 12

WE'VE ALL BEEN ACTING CRAZY

And now I'll return to the Albert Einstein quote introduced at the start of this report:

"INSANITY IS DOING THE SAME THING OVER AND OVER AND *EXPECTING A DIFFERENT RESULT.*"

-ALBERT EINSTEIN

THE FALLACY OF OUR PRACTICE

What have we been doing? We have many patients who we've approached in the same way over and over again, hoping that, one day, they'll suddenly enter our office, miraculously cured! Insanity, for sure!

And I'm not innocent of this mistake, of this blind trust in the methods I've learned and the education I've received.

I've been guilty of it all, too.

But we can no longer do that. I have knowledge, you have knowledge—

WE, TOGETHER, HAVE A *NEW* KNOWLEDGE

—that we are obligated to use toward improving the health of our patients in a more lasting way than traditional chiropractic treatment has been able to achieve.

We have to start using all our resources, not just those we were fed in chiropractic school. We will still look at the postural system, yes, but we'll integrate an acute attention to other disease processes, other organic problems, and other problems in the bodily system as a whole that we can successfully address without need for specialized training or a change in occupation.

Once you start taking a broader view to your patients' health and well-being, everything will change: your patients' outcomes, your connection to your life's work, the success of your practice. *Like mine, your practice will soar.* It will grow. People will seek you out.

And I can testify to all of it. My patients' trust in me has increased and, from that, they regularly refer their friends and family (and strangers!) to me for treatment. My practice has grown. In my personal life, I've seen my mother's health improve tremendously due to a better understanding of what the brain does and how it interacts with the postural system.

> ONCE YOU START TAKING
> A BROADER VIEW
> **EVERYTHING WILL**
> **CHANGE**

Finally, I know solidly that we, chiropractors, are ideally positioned to jumpstart incredible changes in the brain.

And that's a huge leap forward from insanity.

CHAPTER 13

BRAIN CHECK

FOR YOU

As closing to this report, I'd like to ask that you watch this video, "Two Minute Brain Exam for Back Problems" *(URL: http:// ic.instantcustomer.com/go/112834)*, to look at a basic, two-minute neurological examination procedure. On the website, I'll take a couple of minutes to go through the whole examination, explain what certain symptoms mean, and how you can incorporate this procedure with all of your patients in under three minutes.

FOR ME

I've given this report a lot of thought and would like to know what you think. If you are able, please take a few moments to give some feedback and ask me lingering questions about brain-related processes and treatments, addressed or not, in this report, by writing to:

Arjan@BrainCareforChiropractors.com

From the bottom of my heart, I thank you for taking the time to read this report. It's been an urgent and constant ambition for me and, with it and with your help, **we can make that first and critical step toward changing how the world sees chiropractic health care.**

MEDICAL REFERENCES & RESEARCH

INCIDENCE OF BRAIN DECLINE

Olesen J, Leonardi M. *The burden of brain diseases in Europe.* Eur J Neurol. Sept 2003;10(5):471-7.

Olesen J, Gustavsson A, Svenssond M, Wittchene H-U, and Jönsson B on behalf of the CDBE2010 study group and the European Brain Council. *The economic cost of brain disorders in Europe.* European Journal of Neurology 2012; 19: 155-162.

Mayeux R, Stern Y. *Epidemiology of Alzheimer's disease.* Cold Spring HarbPerspect Med. 2012 Aug 1;2(8).

BACK PAIN AND THE BRAIN

Mutso AA1, Petre B, Huang L, Baliki MN, Torbey S, Herrmann KM, Schnitzer TJ, ApkarianAV. *Reorganization of hippocampal functional connectivity with transition to chronic back pain.* JNeurophysiol. 2014 Mar;111(5):1065-76.

Fields HL, Apkarian AV. *Parceling human accumbens into putative core and shell dissociates encoding of values for reward and pain.* JNeurosci. 2013 Oct 9;33(41):16383-93.

Mansour AR, Baliki MN, Huang L, Torbey S, Herrmann KM, Schnitzer TJ, Apkarian AV. *Brain white matter structural properties predict transition to chronic pain.* Pain. 2013 Oct;154(10):2160-8.

CHRONIC PAIN AND THE BRAIN
Committee on Advancing Pain Research, Care, and Education. (2011). *Relieving pain in America: a blueprint for transforming prevention, care, education, and research.* Washington, D.C.: Institute of Medicine of the National Academies.

Cattaneo, A. (2010). *Tanezumab, a recombinant humanized mAb against nerve growth factor for the treatment of acute and chronic pain.* CURRENT OPINION IN MOLECULAR THERAPEUTICS, 12(1), 94–106.

Katz, N., Borenstein, D. G., Birbara, C., Bramson, C., Nemeth, M. A., Smith, M. D., & Brown, M. T. (2011). *Efficacy and safety of tanezumab in the treatment of chronic low back pain.* PAIN, 152(10), 2248–2258.

Kehlet, H., Jensen, T. S., & Woolf, C. J. (2006). *Persistent postsurgical pain: Risk factors and prevention.* LANCET, 367(9522), 1618–1625.

Dijkers, M., Bryce, T., &Zanca, J. (2009). *Prevalence of chronic pain after traumatic spinal cord injury: A systematic review.* JOURNAL OF REHABILITATION RESEARCH AND DEVELOPMENT, 46(1), 13–29.

Backonja, M., Beydoun, A., Edwards, K. R., Schwartz, S. L., Fonseca, V., Hes, M., . . . Garofalo, E. (1998). *Gabapentin for the symptomatic treatment of painful neuropathy in patients with diabetes mellitus: A randomized controlled trial.* JAMA: THE JOURNAL OF THE AMERICAN MEDICAL ASSOCIATION, 280(21), 1831–1836.

May, A. (2011). *Structural brain imaging: A window into chronic pain.* THE NEUROSCIENTIST, 17(2), 209–220.

Seminowicz, D. A., Laferriere, A. L., Millecamps, M., Yu, J. S., Coderre, T. J., & Bushnell, M. C. (2009). *MRI structural brain changes* associated with sensory and emotional function in a rat model of long-term neuropathic pain. NEUROIMAGE, 47(3), 1007–1014.

Baliki, M. N., Schnitzer, T. J., Bauer, W. R., & Apkarian, A. V. (2011). *Brain morphological signatures for chronic pain.* PLOS ONE, 6(10), e26010.

Geha, P. Y., Baliki, M. N., Harden, R. N., Bauer, W. R., Parrish, T. B., & Apkarian, A. V. (2008). *The brain in chronic CRPS pain: Abnormal gray-white matter interactions in emotional and autonomic regions.* NEURON, 60(4), 570–581.

Blum, K., Gardner, E., Oscar-Berman, M., & Gold, M. (2012). *"Liking" and "wanting" linked to Reward Deficiency Syndrome (RDS): Hypothesizing differential responsivity in brain reward circuitry.* CURRENT PHARMACEUTICAL DESIGN, 18(1), 113-118.

Borsook, D., Becerra, L., & Hargreaves, R. (2011). *Biomarkers for chronic pain and analgesia. Part 2: How, where, and what to look for using functional imaging.* DISCOVERY MEDICINE, 11(58), 209–219.

Borsook, D., Becerra, L., & Hargreaves, R. (2011). *Biomarkers for chronic pain and analgesia. Part 1: The need, reality, challenges, and solutions.* DISCOVERY MEDICINE, 11(58), 197–207.

Costigan, M., Belfer, I., Griffin, R. S., Dai, F., Barrett, L. B., Coppola, G., . . . Woolf, C. J. (2010). *Multiple chronic pain states are associated with a common amino acid-changing allele in KCNS1.* BRAIN, 133(9), 2519–2527.

Young, E. E., Lariviere, W. R., & Belfer, I. (2012). *Genetic basis of pain variability: Recent advances.* JOURNAL OF MEDICAL GENETICS, 49(1), 1–9.

Mogil, J. S. (2012). *Pain genetics: Past, present and future.* TRENDS IN GENETICS.

Denk, F., & McMahon, S. B. (2012). *Chronic pain: Emerging evidence for the involvement of epigenetics.* NEURON, 73(3), 435–444.

Tegeder, I., Costigan, M., Griffin, R. S., Abele, A., Belfer, I., Schmidt, H., . . . Woolf, C. J. (2006). *GTP cyclohydrolase and tetrahydrobiopterin regulate pain sensitivity and persistence.* NATURE MEDICINE, 12(11), 1269–1277.

Argoff, C. E. (2010). *Clinical implications of opioid pharmacogenetics.* CLINICAL JOURNAL OF PAIN, 26 SUPPL 10, S16–20.

Jannetto, P. J., & Bratanow, N. C. (2011). *Pain management in the 21st century: Utilization of pharmacogenomics and therapeutic drug monitoring.* EXPERT OPINION ON DRUG METABOLISM AND TOXICOLOGY, 7(6), 745–752.

deVries, B., Frants, R. R., Ferrari, M. D., & van den Maagdenberg, A. M. (2009). *Molecular genetics of migraine.* HUMAN GENETICS, 126(1), 115–132.

Lafreniere, R. G., Cader, M. Z., Poulin, J. F., Andres-Enguix, I., Simoneau, M., Gupta, N., . . . Rouleau, G. A. (2010). *A dominant-negative mutation in the TRESK potassium channel is linked to familial migraine with aura.* NATURE MEDICINE, 16(10), 1157–1160.

Fischer, T. Z., & Waxman, S. G. (2010). *Familial pain syndromes from mutations of the NaV1.7 sodium channel.* ANNALS OF THE NEW YORK ACADEMY OF SCIENCES, 1184, 196–207.

Heinzmann, S., & McMahon, S. B. (2011). *New molecules for the treatment of pain.* CURRENT OPINION IN SUPPORTIVE AND PALLIATIVE CARE, 5(2), 111–1115.

Lotsch, J., & Geisslinger, G. (2011). *Pharmacogenetics of new analgesics.* BRITISH JOURNAL OF PHARMACOLOGY, 163(3), 447–460.

Alexanian, A. R., Svendsen, C. N., Crowe, M. J., & Kurpad, S. N. (2011). *Transplantation of human glial-restricted neural precursors into injured spinal cord promotes functional and sensory recovery without causing allodynia.* CYTOTHERAPY, 13(1), 61–68.

Jain, K. K. (2008). *Gene therapy for pain.* EXPERT OPINION ON BIOLOGICAL THERAPY, 8(12), 1855–1866.

Ren, K., & Dubner, R. (2010). *Interactions between the immune and nervous systems in pain.* NATURE MEDICINE, 16(11), 1267–1276.

Skaper, S. D., Giusti, P., & Facci, L. (2012). *Microglia and mast cells: Two tracks on the road to neuroinflammation.* FASEB JOURNAL.

Banati, R. B., Cagnin, A., Brooks, D. J., Gunn, R. N., Myers, R., Jones, T., . . . Anand, P. (2001). *Long-term trans-synaptic glial responses in the human thalamus after peripheral nerve injury.* NEUROREPORT, 12(16), 3439–3442.

Austin, P. J., &Moalem-Taylor, G. (2010). *The neuro-immune balance in neuropathic pain: Involvement of inflammatory immune cells, immune-like glial cells and cytokines.* JOURNAL OF NEUROIMMUNOLOGY, 229(1–2), 26–50.

Bhutta, A. T., Schmitz, M. L., Swearingen, C., James, L. P., Wardbegnoche, W. L., Lindquist, D. M., . . . Anand, K. J. (2011). *Ketamine as a neuroprotective and anti-inflammatory agent in children undergoing surgery on cardiopulmonary bypass: A pilot randomized, double-blind, placebo-controlled trial.* PEDIATRIC CRITICAL CARE MEDICINE.

Loix, S., De Kock, M., & Henin, P. (2011). *The anti-inflammatory effects of ketamine: State of the Art.* ACTAANAESTHESIOLOGICABELGICA, 62(1), 47–58.

Lamont, K., Chin, M., & Kogan, M. (2011). *Mirror box therapy: Seeing is believing.* EXPLORE, 7(6), 369-372.

Ramachandran, V. S. (2005). *Plasticity and functional recovery in neurology.* CLINICAL MEDICINE, 5(4), 368–373.

Wodlinger, B., & Durand, D. M. (2010). *Peripheral nerve signal recording and processing for artificial limb control.* CONFERENCE PROCEEDINGS OF THE ANNUAL INTERNATIONAL CONFERENCE OF THE

IEEE ENGINEERING IN MEDICINE AND BIOLOGY SOCIETY, 2010, 6206–6209.

Hogan, N., & Krebs, H. I. (2011). *Physically interactive robotic technology for neuromotor rehabilitation.* PROGRESS IN BRAIN RESEARCH, 192, 59–68.

Plow, E. B., Pascual-Leone, A., & Machado, A. (2012). *Brain stimulation in the treatment of chronic neuropathic and non-cancerous pain.* JOURNAL OF PAIN.

Flor, H., & Diers, M. (2009). *Sensorimotor training and cortical reorganization.* NEUROREHABILITATION, 25(1), 19–27.

DeLoach, L. J., Higgins, M. S., Caplan, A. B., & Stiff, J. L. (1998). *The visual analog scale in the immediate postoperative period: Intrasubject variability and correlation with a numeric scale.* ANESTHESIA AND ANALGESIA, 86(1), 102–106.

Nielsen, C. S., Staud, R., & Price, D. D. (2009). *Individual differences in pain sensitivity: Measurement, causation, and consequences.* JOURNAL OF PAIN, 10(3), 231–237.

Coghill, R. C. (2010). *Individual differences in the subjective experience of pain: New insights into mechanisms and models.* HEADACHE, 50(9), 1531–1535.

BRAIN-POSTURE CONNECTION

K. Kamitani, T. Michikawa, S. Iwasawa, N. Eto, T. Tanaka, T. Takebayashi, Y. Nishiwaki. *Spinal Posture in the Sagittal Plane Is Associated With Future Dependence in Activities of Daily Living: A Community-Based Cohort Study of Older Adults in Japan.* The Journals of Gerontology Series A: Biological Sciences and Medical Sciences, 2013.

BRAIN DECLINE & SMELL

Jennifer J. Stamps, Linda M. Bartoshuk, Kenneth M. Heilman. *A brief olfactory test for Alzheimer's disease.* Journal of the Neurological Sciences, 2013; 333 (1-2): 19.

BRAIN DECLINE & BALANCE

A. Kheradmand, A. Lasker, D. S. Zee. *Transcranial Magnetic Stimulation (TMS) of the Supramarginal Gyrus: A Window to Perception of Upright.* Cerebral Cortex, 2013.

BRAIN DECLINE & GAIT

Ervin Sejdic, Kristin Lowry, Jennica Roche, Mark Redfern, Jennifer Brach. *A Comprehensive Assessment of Gait Accelerometry Signals in Time, Frequency and Time-Frequency Domains.* IEEE Transactions on Neural Systems and Rehabilitation Engineering, 2013.

Mielke MM, Roberts RO, Savica R, Cha R, Drubach DI, Christianson T, Pankratz VS, Geda YE, Machulda MM, Ivnik RJ, Knopman DS, Boeve BF, Rocca WA, Petersen RC. *Assessing the temporal relationship between cognition and gait: slow gait predicts cognitive decline in the Mayo Clinic Study of Aging.* JGerontol A BiolSci Med Sci. 2013 Aug;68(8):929-37.

Bridenbaugh SA, Beauchet O, Annweiler C, Allali G, Herrmann F, Kressig RW. *Association between dual task-related decrease in walking speed and real versus imagined Timed Up and Go test performance.* Aging ClinExp Res. 2013 Jun;25(3):283-9.

Caterina Rosano, Howard Aizenstein, Jennifer Brach, Allison Longenberger, Stephanie Studenski, Anne B. Newman. *Gait Measures Indicate Underlying Focal Gray Matter Atrophy in the Brain of Older Adults.* J Gerontol A BiolSci Med Sci. Author manuscript; available in PMC 2009 February 27.Published in final edited form as: J Gerontol A BiolSci Med Sci. 2008 December; 63(12): 1380–1388.

BRAIN ACTIVATION

Appelberg B. *Localization of focal potentials evoked in the red nucleus and ventrolateral nucleus of the thalamus by electrical stimulation of the cerebellar nuclei.* ActaPhysiolScand 1961; 51: 356–70.

Baker J, Gibson A, Glickstein M, Stein J. *Visual cells in the pontine nuclei of the cat.* J Physiol (Lond) 1976; 255: 415–33.

Bodis-Wollner I, Bucher SF, Seelos KC, Paulus W, Reiser M, Oertel WH. *Functional MRI mapping of occipital and frontal cortical activity during voluntary and imagined saccades.* Neurology 1997; 49: 416–20.

Brandt T, Dieterich M. *Pathological eye–head coordination in roll: tonic ocular tilt reaction in mesencephalic and medullary lesions.* Brain 1987; 110: 649–66.

Carpenter MB. *Vestibular nuclei: afferent and efferent projections.* [Review]. Prog Brain Res 1988; 76: 5–15.

Chambers WW, Sprague JM. *Functional localization in the cerebellum. I. Organization in longitudinal cortico-nuclear zones and their contribution to the control of posture, both extrapyramidal and pyramidal.* J Comp Neurol 1955; 103: 105–29.

Clarke S, Miklossy J. *Occipital cortex in man: organization of callosal connections, related myelo- and cytoarchitecture, and putative boundaries of functional visual areas.* J Comp Neurol 1990; 298: 188–214.

Cohen MS, Kosslyn SM, Breiter HC, DiGirolamo GJ, Thompson WL, Anderson AK, et al. *Changes in cortical activity during mental rotation. A mapping study using functional MRI.* Brain 1996; 119: 89–100.

Colebatch JG, Deiber MP, Passingham RE, Friston KJ, Frackowiak RS. *Regional cerebral blood flow during voluntary arm and hand movements in human subjects.* J Neurophysiol 1991; 65: 1392–401.

Courchesne E, Press GA, Murakami J, Berthoty D, Grafe M, Wiley CA, et al. *The cerebellum in sagittal plane–anatomic–MR correlation: the vermis.* Am J Roentgenol 1989; 153: 829–35.

Courville J. *Somatotopical organization of the projection from the nucleus interpositus anterior of the cerebellum to the red nucleus: An experimental study in the cat with silver impregnation methods.* Exp Brain Res 1966; 2: 191–215.

Day BL, Steiger MJ, Thompson PD, Marsden CD. *Effect of vision and stance width on human body motion when standing: implications for afferent control of lateral sway.* J Physiol (Lond) 1993; 469: 479–99.

Diener HC, Dichgans J, Guschlbauer B, Mau H. *The significance of proprioception on postural stabilization as assessed by ischemia.* Brain Res 1984; 296: 103–9.

Diener HC, Dichgans J, Guschlbauer B, Bacher M. *Role of visual and static vestibular influences on dynamic posture control.* Hum Neurobiol 1986; 5: 105–13.

Diener HC, Dichgans J, Guschlbauer B, Bacher M, Langenbach P. *Disturbances of motor preparation in basal ganglia and cerebellar disorders.* Prog Brain Res 1989; 80: 481–8.

Eager RP. *Efferent cortico-nuclear pathways in the cerebellum of the cat.* J Comp Neurol 1963; 120: 81–103.

Fife TD, Baloh RW. *Disequilibrium of unknown cause in older people.* Ann Neurol 1993; 34: 694–702.

Flumerfelt BA, Otabe S, Courville J. *Distinct projections to the red nucleus from the dentate and interposed nuclei in the monkey.* Brain Res 1973; 50: 408–14.

Friston KJ, Ashburner J, Frith CD, Poline JP, Heather JD, Frackowiak RSJ. *Spatial registration and normalization of images.* Hum Brain Mapp 1995a; 3: 165–89.

Friston KJ, Holmes AP, Worsley KJ, Poline JP, Frith CD, Frackowiak RS. *Statistical parametric mapping in functional imaging: a general linear approach.* Hum Brain Mapp 1995b; 2: 189–210.

Fukuyama H, Ouchi Y, Matsuzaki S, Nagahama Y, Yamauchi H, Ogawa M, et al. *Brain functional activity during gait in normal subjects: a SPECT study.* NeurosciLett 1997; 228: 183–6.

Haerer AF. *DeJong's the neurologic examination.* 5th edn. Philadelphia: J.B. Lippincott; 1992.

Holmes G. *The Croonian Lectures on the clinical symptoms of cerebellar disease, and their interpretation.* Lancet 1922a; 1: 1177–82, 1231–7.

Holmes G. The Croonian Lectures on the clinical symptoms of cerebellar disease, and their interpretation. Lancet 1922b; 2: 59–65, 111–5.

Horak FB, Shumway-Cook A, Crowe TK, Black FO. *Vestibular function and motor proficiency of children with impaired hearing, or with learning disability and motor impairments.* Dev Med Child Neurol 1988; 30: 64–79.

Horak FB, Nashner LM, Diener HC. *Postural strategies associated with somatosensory and vestibular loss.* Exp Brain Res 1990; 82: 167–77.

Ito M. *The cerebellum and neural control.* New York: Raven; 1984.

Ivry RB, Keele SW, Diener HC. *Dissociation of the lateral and medial cerebellum in movement timing and movement execution.* Exp Brain Res 1988; 73: 167–80.

Koller WC, Wilson RS, Glatt SL, Huckman MS, Fox JR. *Senile gait: correlation with computed tomographic scans* [letter]. Ann Neurol 1983; 13: 343–4.

Kotchabhakdi N, Walberg F. *Primary vestibular afferent projections to the cerebellum as demonstrated by retrograde axonal transport of horseradish peroxidase.* Brain Res 1978; 142: 142–6.

Lassen NA, Roland PE, Larsen B, Melamed E, Soh K. *Mapping of human cerebral functions: a study of the regional cerebral blood flow pattern during rest, its reproducibility and the activations seen during basic sensory and motor functions.* ActaNeurolScandSuppl 1977; 64: 262–3.

Leicht R, Schmidt RF. *Somatotopic studies on the vermal cortex of the cerebellar anterior lobe of unanesthetized cats.* Exp Brain Res 1977; 27: 479–90.

Leicht R, Rowe MJ, Schmidt RF. *Mossy and climbing fiber inputs from cutaneous mechanoreceptors to cerebellar Purkinje cells in unanesthetized cats.* Exp Brain Res 1977; 27: 451–77.

Lord SR, Clark RD, Webster IW. *Postural stability and associated physiological factors in a population of aged persons.* J Gerontol 1991; 46: M69–76.

McKeefry DJ, Watson JD, Frackowiak RS, Fong K, Zeki S. *The activity in human areas V1/V2, V3, and V5 during the perception of coherent and incoherent motion.* Neuroimage 1997; 5: 1–12.

Miller S, Van Der Burg J, Van Der Meche F. *Coordination of movements of the hindlimbs and forelimbs in different forms of locomotion in normal and decerebrate cats.* Brain Res 1975; 91: 217–37.

Mitchell J. *Postural reactions of the lower limb to centre-of-gravity displacements in one-foot stance.* Physiotherapy 1971; 57: 562–70.

Nagahama Y, Takayama Y, Fukuyama H, Yamauchi H, Matsuzaki S, Magata Y, et al. *Functional anatomy on perception of position and motion in depth.* Neuroreport 1996; 7: 1717–21.

Nashner LM. *Adapting reflexes controlling the human posture.* Exp Brain Res 1976; 26: 59–72.

Nashner LM, Black FO, Wall C 3rd. *Adaptation to altered support and visual conditions during stance: patients with vestibular deficits.* J Neurosci 1982; 2: 536–44.

Nitschke MF, Kleinschmidt A, Wessel K, Frahm J. *Somatotopic motor representation in the human anterior cerebellum. A high-resolution functional MRI study.* Brain 1996; 119: 1023–9.

Norre ME, Forrez G, Beckers A. *Vestibular dysfunction causing instability in aged patients.* ActaOtolaryngol (Stockh) 1987; 104: 50–5.

Ouchi Y, Nobesawa S, Okada H, Yoshikawa E, Futatsubashi M, Kanako M. *Glucose metabolism of the human hippocampal formation in the hippocampal long axis plane measured by PET.* J Cereb Blood Flow Metab 1997; 17 Suppl: S218.

Parent A. *Human Neuroanatomy.* 9th edn. Baltimore: Williams and Wilkins; 1996.

Paus T. *Location and function of the human frontal eye-field: a selective review.* [Review]. Neuropsychologia 1996; 34: 475–83.

Ptito A, Zatorre RJ, Petrides M, Frey S, Alivisatos B, Evans AC. *Localization and lateralization of stereoscopic processing in the human brain.* Neuroreport 1993; 4: 1155–8.

Raichle ME, Martin WR, Herscovitch P, Mintun MA, Markham J. *Brain blood flow measured with intravenous H2(15)O. II. Implementation and validation.* J Nucl Med 1983; 24: 790–8.

Richardson JK, Ashton-Miller JA, Lee SG, Jacobs K. *Moderate peripheral neuropathy impairs weight transfer and unipedal balance in the elderly.* Arch Phys Med Rehabil 1996; 77: 1152–6.

Roland PE, Larsen B, Lassen NA, Skinhoj E. *Supplementary motor area and other cortical areas in organization of voluntary movements in man.* J Neurophysiol 1980; 43: 118–36.

Talairach J, Tournoux P. *Co-planar stereotaxic atlas of the human brain: 3-dimensional proportional system: an approach to cerebral imaging.* Stuttgart: Thieme; 1988.

Tolbert DL, Bantli H, Bloedel JR. *Multiple branching of cerebellar efferent projections in cats.* Exp Brain Res 1978; 31: 305–16.

Waespe W, Cohen B, Raphan T. *Dynamic modification of the vestibulo-ocular reflex by the nodulus and uvula.* Science 1985; 228: 199–202.

Wessel K, Nitschke MF. *Cerebellar somatotopic representation and cerebro-cerebellar interconnections in ataxic patients.* Prog Brain Res 1997; 114: 577–88.

Wolfson L, Whipple MA, Derby CA, Amerman P, Murphy T, Tobin JN, et al. *A dynamic posturography study of balance in healthy elderly.* Neurology 1992; 42: 2069–75.

Yamashita T, Uchida H, Okada H, Kurono T, Takemori T, Watanabe M, et al. *Development of a high resolution PET.* IEEE Trans NuclSci 1990; 37: 594–9.

THE BRAIN AND THE EFFECTS OF HEAD INJURY

Josef M. Ling, Stefan Klimaj, Trent Toulouse, and Andrew R. Mayer. *A prospective study of gray matter abnormalities in mild traumatic brain injury.* Neurology, November 2013.

Tanya Charyk Stewart, Jason Gilliland, Douglas D. Fraser. *An epidemiologic profile of pediatric concussions.* Journal of Trauma and Acute Care Surgery, 2014; 76 (3): 736.

Adibhatla, R. M., & Hatcher, J. F. (2008). *Altered lipid metabolism in brain injury and disorders.* Sub-cellular Biochemistry, 49, 241–268.

Mellick, D., Gerhart, K. A., & Whiteneck, G. G. (2003). *Understanding outcomes based on the post-acute hospitalization pathways followed by persons with traumatic brain injury.* Brain Injury, 17(1), 55–71.

Gomez-Pinilla, F., Ying, Z., Roy, R. R., Molteni, R., & Edgerton, V. R. (2002). *Voluntary exercise induces a BDNF-mediated mechanism that promotes neuroplasticity.* Journal of Neurophysiology, 88(5), 2187–2195.

Gomez-Pinilla, F. (Ed.). (2010). *The Therapeutic Potential of Diet and Exercise on Brain Repair* (3rd ed.). Boca Raton, FL: CRC Press, Taylor & Francis Group.

Ashley, M. J., Weintraub, A., & Ripley, D. (2010). *Bioscience frontiers in neuromedical intervention following brain injury.* In M. J. Ashley

(Ed.), Traumatic Brain Injury: Rehabilitation, Treatment and Case Management (pp. 419–454). Boca Raton: CRC Press, Taylor & Francis Group.

High, W. M., Briones-Galang, M., Clark, J. A., Gilkison, C., Mossberg, K. A., Zgaljardic, D. J., . . . Urban, R. J. (2010). *Effect of growth hormone therapy on cognition after traumatic brain injury.* Journal of Neurotrauma, 27, 1565–1575.

Gauthier, L. V. M. A., Taub, E. P., Perkins, C. B. S., Ortmann, M., Mark, V. W. M. D., & Uswatte, G. P. (2008). *Remodeling the brain: Plastic structural brain changes produced by different motor therapies after stroke.* Stroke, 39(5), 1520–1525.

Shiel, A., Burn, J. P., Henry, D., Clark, J., Wilson, B. A., Burnett, M. E., & McLellan, D. L. (2001). *The effects of increased rehabilitation therapy after brain injury: results of a prospective controlled trial.* Clinical Rehabilitation, 15(5), 501–514.

Spivack, G., Spettell, C. M., Ellis, D. W., & Ross, S. E. (1992). *Effects of intensity of treatment and length of stay on rehabilitation.* Brain Injury, 6(5), 419–434.

Zhu, X. L., Poon, W. S., Chan, C. H., & Chan, S. H. (2001). *Does intensive rehabilitation change the functional outcome of patients with traumatic brain injury? Interim result of a randomized controlled trial.* British Journal of Neurosurgery, 15(6), 464–473.

BRAIN & COGNITION

Llinás RR. *The olivo-cerebellar system: a key to understanding the functional significance of intrinsic oscillatory brain properties.* Front Neural Circuits. 2014 Jan 28; 7:96.

TESTING OF THE BRAIN

Q. Arshad, Y. Nigmatullina, A. M. Bronstein. *Handedness-Related Cortical Modulation of the Vestibular-Ocular Reflex.* Journal of Neuroscience, 2013; 33 (7): 3221.

ONE-LEGGED BALANCE TEST
Yves Rolland, Gabor Abellan van Kan, FatiNourhashemi, Sandrine Andrieu, ChristelleCantet, Sophie Guyonnet-Gillette and Bruno Vellas. *An Abnormal 'One-leg Balance' Test Predicts Cognitive Decline During Alzheimer's Disease.* Journal of Alzheimer's Disease, 16:3 March 2009.

EYES AND POSTURE
S. Glasauer, PhD, E. Schneider, PhD, K. Jahn, MD, M. Strupp, MD and T.Brandt, MD. *How the eyes move the body.* Neurology October 25, 2005 vol. 65 no. 8 1291-1293.

CURCUMIN (A.K.A. TURMERIC)
Jung KK, Lee HS, Cho JY, Shin WC, Rhee MH, Kim TG, Kang JH, Kim SH, Hong S, Kang SY. *Inhibitory effect of curcumin on nitric oxide production from lipopolysaccharide-activated primary microglia.* Life Sci. 2006 Oct 19;79(21):2022-31.

Yang S1, Zhang D, Yang Z, Hu X, Qian S, Liu J, Wilson B, Block M, Hong JS. *Curcumin protects dopaminergic neuron against LPS induced neurotoxicity in primary rat neuron/glia culture.* Neurochem Res. 2008 Oct; 33(10): 2044-53. doi: 10.1007/s11064-008-9675-z.

MAGNESIUM
Crowther CA, Hiller JE, Doyle LW, Haslam RR; *Australasian Collaborative Trial of Magnesium Sulphate* (ACTOMg SO4) Collaborative Group.

Effect of magnesium sulfate given for neuroprotection before preterm birth: a randomized controlled trial. JAMA. 2003 Nov 26;290(20):2669-76.

New experimental and clinical data on the efficacy of pharmacological magnesium infusions in cerebral infarcts. Muir KW. Magnes Res. 1998 Mar;11(1):43-56. Review.

GLUTHATIONE

Tewthanom K1, Janwityanuchit S, Totemchockchyakarn K, Panomvana D. *Correlation of lipid peroxidation and glutathione levels with severity of systemic lupus erythematosus: a pilot study from single centre.* J Pharm Pharm Sci. 2008;11(3):30-4.

Yan Z, Banerjee R. *Redox remodeling as an immunoregulatory strategy.* Biochemistry. 2010 Feb 16;49(6):1059-66. doi: 10.1021/bi902022n. Review.

VITAMIN D

Singh A, Kamen DL. *Potential benefits of vitamin D for patients with systemic lupus erythematosus.* Dermatoendocrinol. 2012 Apr 1;4(2):146-51.

Antico A, Tampoia M, Tozzoli R, Bizzaro N. *Can supplementation with vitamin D reduce the risk or modify the course of autoimmune diseases? A systematic review of the literature.* Autoimmun Rev. 2012 Dec; 12(2):127-36.

ALPHA-LIPOIC ACID

Konrad T, Vicini P, Kusterer K, Höflich A, Assadkhani A, Böhles HJ, Sewell A, Tritschler HJ, Cobelli C, Usadel KH. *Alpha-Lipoic acid treatment decreases serum lactate and pyruvate concentrations and improves glucose effectiveness in lean and obese patients with type 2 diabetes.* Diabetes Care. 1999 Feb; 22(2):280-7.

Nagamatsu M, Nickander KK, Schmelzer JD, Raya A, Wittrock DA, Tritschler H, Low PA. *Lipoic acid improves nerve blood flow, reduces oxidative stress, and improves distal nerve conduction in experimental diabetic neuropathy.* Diabetes Care. 1995 Aug;18(8):1160-7.

L-CARNITINE

Greco AV, Mingrone G, Bianchi M, Ghirlanda G. *Effect of propionyl-L-carnitine in the treatment of diabetic angiopathy: controlled double blind trial versus placebo.* Drugs ExpClin Res. 1992;18(2):69-80.

ALPHA GPC

Lopez CM, Govoni S, Battaini F, Bergamaschi S, Longoni A, Giaroni C, Trabucchi M. *Effect of a new cognition enhancer, alpha-glycerylphosphorylcholine, on scopolamine-induced amnesia and brain acetylcholine.* PharmacolBiochemBehav. 1991 Aug;39(4):835-40.

Sigala S1, Imperato A, Rizzonelli P, Casolini P, Missale C, Spano P. *L-alpha-glycerylphosphorylcholine antagonizes scopolamine-induced amnesia and enhances hippocampal cholinergic transmission in the rat.* Eur J Pharmacol. 1992 Feb 18;211(3):351-8.

PHOSPHATIDYL SERINE

Crook TH1, Tinklenberg J, Yesavage J, Petrie W, Nunzi MG, Massari DC. *Effects of phosphatidylserine in age-associated memory impairment.* Neurology. 1991 May;41(5):644-9.

OMEGA 3

J. V. Pottala, K. Yaffe, J. G. Robinson, M. A. Espeland, R. Wallace, W. S. Harris. *Higher RBC EPA DHA corresponds with larger total brain and hippocampal volumes: WHIMS-MRI Study.* Neurology, 2014.

Z. S. Tan, W. S. Harris, A. S. Beiser, R. Au, J. J. Himali, S. Debette, A. Pikula, C. DeCarli, P. A. Wolf, R. S. Vasan, S. J. Robins, S. Seshadri. *Red blood cell omega-3 fatty acid levels and markers of accelerated brain aging.* Neurology, 2012; 78 (9): 658.

HUPERZINE

Zhao HW, Li XY. *Ginkgolide A, B, and huperzine A inhibit nitric oxide-induced neurotoxicity.* IntImmunopharmacol. 2002 Oct;2(11):1551-6.

Pavlov VA1, Parrish WR, Rosas-Ballina M, Ochani M, Puerta M, Ochani K, Chavan S, Al-Abed Y, Tracey KJ. *Brain acetylcholinesterase activity controls systemic cytokine levels through the cholinergic anti-inflammatory pathway.* Brain Behav Immun. 2009 Jan;23(1):41-5.

Vinpocitine

Souness JE1, Brazdil R, Diocee BK, Jordan R. *Role of selective cyclic GMP phosphodiesterase inhibition in the myorelaxant actions of M&B 22,948, MY-5445, vinpocetine and 1-methyl-3-isobutyl-8-(methylamino) xanthine.* Br J Pharmacol. 1989 Nov;98(3):725-34.

Evgenov OV1, Busch CJ, Evgenov NV, Liu R, Petersen B, Falkowski GE, Petho B, Vas A, Bloch KD, Zapol WM, Ichinose F. *Inhibition of phosphodiesterase 1 augments the pulmonary vasodilator response to inhaled nitric oxide in awake lambs with acute pulmonary hypertension.* Am J Physiol Lung Cell Mol Physiol. 2006 Apr;290(4):L723-L729. Epub 2005 Nov 11.

Gingko Biloba

Jezova D1, Duncko R, Lassanova M, Kriska M, Moncek F. *Reduction of rise in blood pressure and cortisol release during stress by Ginkgo biloba extract (EGb 761) in healthy volunteers.* J PhysiolPharmacol. 2002 Sep;53(3):337-48.

Umegaki K, Shinozuka K, Watarai K, Takenaka H, Yoshimura M, Daohua P, EsashiT. *Ginkgobiloba extract attenuates the development of hypertension in deoxycorticosterone acetate-salt hypertensive rats.* ClinExpPharmacol Physiol. 2000 Apr;27(4):277-82.

Bacopa Monieri

Roodenrys S1, Booth D, Bulzomi S, Phipps A, Micallef C, Smoker J. *Chronic effects of Brahmi (Bacopamonnieri) on human memory.* Neuropsychopharmacology. 2002 Aug;27(2):279-81.

Calabrese C1, Gregory WL, Leo M, Kraemer D, Bone K, Oken B. *Effects of a standardized Bacopamonnieri extract on cognitive performance, anxiety, and depression in the elderly: a randomized, double-blind, placebo-controlled trial.* J Altern Complement Med. 2008 Jul;14(6):707-13.

Sleep

Siegel J M. *The REM Sleep-Memory Consolidation Hypothesis,* Science 2001 (vol. 294, November): 1058-1063.

Backhaus J, et al. *Midlife decline in declarative memory consolidation is correlated with a decline in slow wave sleep*, Learning and Memory 2007 (vol. 14): 336-341.

Lim A S, et al. *Increased fragmentation of rest-activity patterns is associated with a characteristic pattern of cognitive impairment in older individuals*, Sleep 2012 (May 1): 633-640.

Peigneux P, et al. *Are Spatial Memories Strengthened in the Human Hippocampus during Slow Wave Sleep?* Neuron 2004 (vol. 44, Oct 28): 535—545.

GUT-BRAIN AXIS

Barden, N. (2004). *Implication of the hypothalamic-pituitary-adrenal axis in the physiopathology of depression*. J Psychiatry Neurosci 29, 185-193.

Beaumont, W. (1833). *Experiments and observations on the gastric juice and the physiology of digestion* (Plattsburg: F.P. Allen).

Bech-Nielsen, G.V., Hansen, C.H., Hufeldt, M.R., Nielsen, D.S., Aasted, B., Vogensen, F.K., Midtvedt, T., and Hansen, A.K. (2011). *Manipulation of the gut microbiota in C57BL/6 mice changes glucose tolerance without affecting weight development and gut mucosal immunity.* Res Vet Sci.

Benton, D., Williams, C., and Brown, A. (2007). *Impact of consuming a milk drink containing a probiotic on mood and cognition*. European journal of clinical nutrition 61, 355-361.

Bercik, P., Denou, E., Collins, J., Jackson, W., Lu, J., Jury, J., Deng, Y., Blennerhassett, P., Macri, J., McCoy, K.D., et al. (2011a). *The intestinal microbiota affect central levels of brain-derived neurotropic factor and behavior in mice.* Gastroenterology 141, 599-609, 609 e591-593.

Bercik, P., Park, A.J., Sinclair, D., Khoshdel, A., Lu, J., Huang, X., Deng, Y., Blennerhassett, P.A., Fahnestock, M., Moine, D., et al. (2011b). *The anxiolytic effect of Bifidobacteriumlongum*

NCC3001 *involves vagal pathways for gut-brain communication.* NeurogastroenterolMotil 23, 1132-1139.

Bercik, P., Verdu, E.F., Foster, J.A., Macri, J., Potter, M., Huang, X., Malinowski, P., Jackson, W., Blennerhassett, P., Neufeld, K.A., et al. (2010). *Chronic gastrointestinal inflammation induces anxiety-like behavior and alters central nervous system biochemistry in mice.* Gastroenterology 139, 2102-2112 e2101.

Bravo, J.A., Forsythe, P., Chew, M.V., Escaravage, E., Savignac, H.M., Dinan, T.G., Bienenstock, J., and Cryan, J.F. (2011). *Ingestion of Lactobacillus strain regulates emotional behavior and central GABA receptor expression in a mouse via the vagus nerve.* ProcNatlAcadSci U S A 108, 16050-16055.

Cannon, W.B. (1909). *The influence of emotional states on the functions of the alimentary canal.* Am J Med Sci 137, 480-487.

Clarke, G., Grenham, S., Scully, P., Fitzgerald, P., Moloney, R.D., Shanahan, F., Dinan, T.G., and Cryan, J.F. (2012). *The microbiome-gut-brain axis during early life regulates the hippocampal serotonergic system in a sex-dependent manner.* Mol Psychiatry.

Costello, E.K., Lauber, C.L., Hamady, M., Fierer, N., Gordon, J.I., and Knight, R. (2009). *Bacterial community variation in human body habitats across space and time.* Science 326, 1694-1697.

Desbonnet, L., Garrett, L., Clarke, G., Kiely, B., Cryan, J.F., & Dinan, T.G. (2010). *Effects of the probiotic Bifidobacteriuminfantis in the maternal separation model of depression.* Neuroscience 170, 1179-1188.

Foster, J.A., & McVey Neufeld, K.A. (2013). *Gut-brain axis: how the microbiome influences anxiety and depression.* Trends Neurosci 36, 305-312.

Furness, J.B. (2012). *The enteric nervous system and neurogastroenterology.* Nature reviews Gastroenterology & Hepatology 9, 286-294.

Gareau, M.G., Jury, J., MacQueen, G., Sherman, P.M., & Perdue, M.H. (2007). *Probiotic treatment of rat pups normalisescorticosterone* release and ameliorates colonic dysfunction induced by maternal separation. Gut 56, 1522-1528.

Gareau, M.G., Silva, M.A., & Perdue, M.H. (2008). *Pathophysiological mechanisms of stress-induced intestinal damage.* Current molecular medicine 8, 274-281.

Gill, S.R., Pop, M., Deboy, R.T., Eckburg, P.B., Turnbaugh, P.J., Samuel, B.S., Gordon, J.I., Relman, D.A., Fraser-Liggett, C.M., & Nelson, K.E. (2006). *Metagenomic analysis of the human distal gut microbiome.* Science 312, 1355-1359.

Goehler, L.E., Park, S.M., Opitz, N., Lyte, M., & Gaykema, R.P. (2008). *Campylobacter jejuni infection increases anxiety-like behavior in the holeboard: possible anatomical substrates for viscerosensory modulation of exploratory behavior.* Brain BehavImmun 22, 354-366.

Heijtz, R.D., Wang, S., Anuar, F., Qian, Y., Bjorkholm, B., Samuelsson, A., Hibberd, M.L., Forssberg, H., & Pettersson, S. (2011). *Normal gut microbiota modulates brain development and behavior.* ProcNatlAcadSci U S A 108, 3047-3052.

Hooper, L.V., Wong, M.H., Thelin, A., Hansson, L., Falk, P.G., & Gordon, J.I. (2001). *Molecular analysis of commensal host-microbial relationships in the intestine.* Science 291, 881-884.

Jumpertz, R., Le, D.S., Turnbaugh, P.J., Trinidad, C., Bogardus, C., Gordon, J.I., & Krakoff, J. (2011). *Energy-balance studies reveal associations between gut microbes, caloric load, and nutrient absorption in humans.* Am J ClinNutr 94, 58-65.

Kau, A.L., Ahern, P.P., Griffin, N.W., Goodman, A.L., & Gordon, J.I. (2011). *Human nutrition, the gut microbiome and the immune system.* Nature 474, 327-336.

Lyte, M., Li, W., Opitz, N., Gaykema, R.P., & Goehler, L.E. (2006). *Induction of anxiety-like behavior in mice during the initial stages of infection with the agent of murine colonic hyperplasia Citrobacterrodentium.* PhysiolBehav 89, 350-357.

Macpherson, A.J., & Harris, N.L. (2004). *Interactions between commensal intestinal bacteria and the immune system.* Nat Rev Immunol 4, 478-485.

Messaoudi, M., Violle, N., Bisson, J.F., Desor, D., Javelot, H., & Rougeot, C. (2011). *Beneficial psychological effects of a probiotic formulation (Lactobacillus helveticus R0052 and Bifidobacteriumlongum R0175) in healthy human volunteers.* Gut microbes 2, 256-261.

Neufeld, K.A., Kang, N., Bienenstock, J., & Foster, J.A. (2011a). *Effects of intestinal microbiota on anxiety-like behavior.* CommunIntegrBiol 4, 492-494.

Neufeld, K.M., Kang, N., Bienenstock, J., & Foster, J.A. (2011b). *Reduced anxiety-like behavior and central neurochemical change in germ-free mice.* NeurogastroenterolMotil 23, 255-264, e119.

Pavlov, I. (1910). *The work of digestive glands.* [English translation from Russian by W. H. Thompson.] (London: Griffen).

Qin, J., Li, R., Raes, J., Arumugam, M., Burgdorf, K.S., Manichanh, C., Nielsen, T., Pons, N., Levenez, F., Yamada, T., et al. (2010). *A human gut microbial gene catalogue established by metagenomic sequencing.* Nature 464, 59-65.

Rao, A.V., Bested, A.C., Beaulne, T.M., Katzman, M.A., Iorio, C., Berardi, J.M., & Logan, A.C. (2009). *A randomized, double-blind, placebo-controlled pilot study of a probiotic in emotional symptoms of chronic fatigue syndrome.* Gut Pathog 1, 6.

Schloissnig, S., Arumugam, M., Sunagawa, S., Mitreva, M., Tap, J., Zhu, A., Waller, A., Mende, D.R., Kultima, J.R., Martin, J., et al. (2013). *Genomic variation landscape of the human gut microbiome.* Nature 493, 45-50.

Serino, M., Chabo, C., & Burcelin, R. (2012). *Intestinal MicrobiOMICS to define health and disease in human and mice.* Current pharmaceutical biotechnology 13, 746-758.

Sudo, N., Chida, Y., Aiba, Y., Sonoda, J., Oyama, N., Yu, X.N., Kubo, C., & Koga, Y. (2004). *Postnatal microbial colonization programs the hypothalamic-pituitary-adrenal system for stress response in mice.* J Physiol 558, 263-275.

Teitelbaum, A.A., Gareau, M.G., Jury, J., Yang, P.C., & Perdue, M.H. (2008). *Chronic peripheral administration of corticotropin-releasing factor causes colonic barrier dysfunction similar to psychological stress.* Am J PhysiolGastrointest Liver Physiol 295, G452-459.

DIET & LIFESTYLE
Hartman AL, Rubenstein JE, Kossoff EH. *Intermittent fasting: A "new" historical strategy for controlling seizures?* Epilepsy Research, J Epilepsy Res 2012.10.011.

Seyfried BT, Kiebish M, Marsh J, Mukherjee P. *Targeting energy metabolism in brain cancer through calorie restriction and the ketogenic diet.* J Can Res Ther 2009;5:7-15.

Stafstrom, CE & Rho JM. *The Ketogenic Diet as a Treatment Paradigm for Diverse Neurological Disorders.* Front Pharmacol 2012; 3:59.

Cunnane S, Nugent S, Roy, M et al. *Brain Fuel metabolism, aging and Alzheimer's Disease.* Nutrition 27 (2011) 3-2.

MEDITATION
Brewer JA, Davis JH, Goldstein J. *Why is it so hard to pay attention, or is it? Mindfulness, the factors of awakening and reward-based learning.* Mindfulness (NY). 2013 Mar 1;4(1).

Brewer JA, Garrison KA, Whitfield-Gabrieli S. *What about the "Self" is Processed in the Posterior Cingulate Cortex?* Front Hum Neurosci. 2013 Oct 2;7:647. eCollection 2013. Review.

Brewer JA, Garrison KA. *The posterior cingulate cortex as a plausible mechanistic target of meditation: findings from neuroimaging.* Ann N Y Acad Sci. 2014 Jan;1307(1):19-27.

STRESS & BRAIN DEVELOPMENT

Joels, M., Pu, Z., Wiegert, O.,Oitzl, M. S., & Krugers, H. J. *Learning under stress: How does it work?* TRENDS IN COGNITIVE SCIENCES, 2006, 10(4), 152–158.

Gentile, D. A., & Stone, W. Violent video game effects on children and adolescents. A review of the literature. MINERVA PEDIATRICA, 2005, 57(6), 337–358.

About the Author

ARJAN KUIPERS,
DC, BSC, DACNB, FACFN, FEAC (NEUROLOGY)

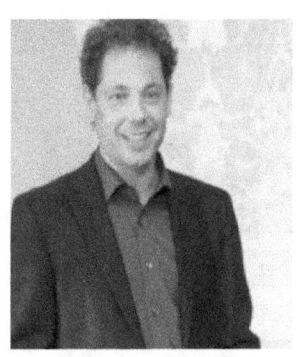

Arjan Kuipers is a chiropractic neurologist and has been a practicing clinician for over two decades. He is the founder and chief innovator of *ADHD & Autism Training* and *Brain Care for Chiropractors*, which provide in-the-know answers for parents and their children with neurodevelopmental disorders, chiropractic professionals, and patients.

Arjan is known for his astute and discriminative way of solving problems and upgrading for future results.

His clinical "TOBE" training has been used with hundreds of children with a diagnosis of ADHD and/or autism. To date, he has helped over 10,000 people improve their situations with his knowledge of the interaction between the postural system and brain.

Arjan has lectured throughout Europe and has shared the stage and his thoughts with many leaders in neurodevelopmental and brain science, including Sally Goddard, author of *Reflexes, Learning and Behavior*; neuroscientist Mike Merzenich; and auditory stimulation expert Kjeld Johansen.

His publications include the *Help! My Child has ADHD/Autism* book series (three volumes), "20 Top Questions Every Parent

Should Ask About ADHD/Autism", and "5 Forgotten Factors that can Make a Difference in the Life of Your Child with ADHD/Autism" (in Dutch).

Originally from the old town of Elburg in the Netherlands, Arjan now lives with Anniken in Zutphen (Netherlands) and Trondheim (Norway); together they have four children. He loves the outdoors, hiking, and is a passionate fly fisher.

Arjan maintains a website (www.arjankuipers.com) and may be contacted at:

Arjan@BrainCareforChiropractors.com

##